Ananda Yoga for Higher Awareness

Swami Kriyananda (J. Donald Walters)

Ananda Yoga for Higher Awareness

Swami Kriyananda (J. Donald Walters)

Crystal Clarity Publishers
Nevada City, California

ISBN: 1-56589-078-7
Printed in the USA
Cover photograph of Swami Kriyananda by Dick Powers
Original cover photography by Swami Kriyananda

Crystal Clarity Publishers
146918 Tyler-Foote Road
Nevada City, CA 95959

800.424.1055 or 530.478.7600
f. 530.478.7610
clarity@crystalclarity.com
www.crystalclarity.com

21 20 19 18 17 16 15

Table of Contents

1

Basic Principles

The Purpose of Yoga Postures

In the main stream of life two currents, especially, may be observed. One is toward an expansion of awareness. The other is a sinking back into sleep and unawareness, a shutting out of reality, a longing for death. Positive and negative—in all of us, both of these trends may be observed.

To the extent that we draw the world to us, by an attitude of willingness, appreciation, kindness, joy, we express the positive current. When, by unwillingness, a critical attitude, selfishness, unkindness, grief, we push the world away from us, excluding it from our circle of awareness, we express the negative current. Man, unlike the lower animals, has the freedom greatly to quicken his evolutional climb toward perfect awareness—or, if he prefers, to fall back into the mires of unknowing from which he emerged. It is for him to rejoice in his existence, or merely to wallow in it.

Every growth in awareness is, in the last analysis, a growth in *Self*-awareness. What we observe in the world depends on our own *capacity* for observation. An anguished spirit will find in everything justification for its anguish. A joyous spirit will see reasons for gladness everywhere. No amount of pious maxims or lofty philosophy can bring light into man's world beyond what already exists in his own consciousness.

The true purpose of yoga is to facilitate the development of this Self-awareness—not as a self-enclosure, but as a doorway to an expanded awareness of the surrounding universe, of truth, of very life.

Usually, hatha yoga (the science of yoga *asanas*, or postures) is taught only from a standpoint of its benefits to the body. And from this standpoint it might well be said that the yoga postures, as a system for achieving longevity and radiant health, stand supreme. We have personally seen old men, practitioners of this science, who might have passed for young men in their thirties. At Allahabad we met an ancient yogi, named Deohara Baba, who was reputed to be 140 years old. His hair was black, his body muscular. He could easily have been taken for a man of about 50.

Old age and sickness settle first in the joints and in the spinal discs. Anatomical studies reveal that these spinal discs often begin to show signs of degeneration as early as man's third decade, which is to say, in his twenties. The yoga postures loosen the joints; they stretch and irrigate the vertebrae, keeping them youthful even late into old age. They promote the free flow of energy throughout the nervous system and assist in the elimination of toxins and poisons from the joints and other body parts where these foreign elements tend otherwise to settle, sometimes permanently. The postures exert a beneficial pressure on various glands and internal organs, flushing and stimulating them. Even a little bit of this practice can produce astonishing improvements in one's general health.

It is small wonder, then, that hatha yoga should be growing in popularity in the West as rapidly as it is. A few years ago an article in California's *Palo Alto Times* (now the *Peninsula Times Tribune*) listed the grievances of high school students in a neighboring community. Among the "rights" demanded by those youngsters was instruction in the yoga postures.

Yes, whether for good or ill, the *asanas* are well on their way to becoming a fad. But the aim of these postures, so far, has generally been recognized to be only the promotion of physical health. Much more is involved.

For by the yoga postures one can improve his mental outlook. He can achieve a richer, more harmonious emotional life. The postures are a definite aid to spiritual development. Particularly, from a standpoint of the approach of this book, they help one to develop a more vital awareness. The hatha yogi (a yogi is one who practices the yoga science) learns to include his body in the general circle of his awareness, to *live* in his body instead

of merely existing in it. By increasing his physical awareness he can free his mind from the imperatives so commonly imposed upon man by his body: weakness, fatigue,
physical sluggishness and resistance, discomfort, pain. He
is thus able to make the body the servant of his will.
Health, as it is usually conceived, is negative: a mere absence of disease. But the yoga postures help to create a
joyous sense of vitality and well-being. They make the
body an ally, not a neutral neighbor or even a foe, of the
soul in its search for expanding awareness.

Physical Postures and Mental Awareness

Certain bodily postures are naturally associated with
certain mental attitudes. When the mind is dis-
couraged, the body tends to stoop forward. Courage tends
to make the body erect. Under the influence of aggressive feelings, the shoulders often become hunched upward, the fists become clenched. When feeling stubborn
a person may jut his jaw forward. When he is inspired,
his eyes will look upward; when depressed, they will look
downward. Poise, or lack of it, is reflected in the way
one sits, in the way he stands, in the movement of his
hands.

Even the pattern of breathing is affected by one's mental attitudes. Fear and anxiety tighten the stomach muscles. A person with a narrow, self-restrictive outlook inclines to draw in the sides of his rib cage. One who suppresses his natural feelings tends to hold in the upper part of his chest. Can a person with all of these psychological problems find any room for breathing at all? Hardly! The amount of oxygen he permits his system amounts to starvation wages, truly.

But just as one's mental attitudes affect his body, so also his bodily postures affect his mind. Slumped shoulders and a bent spine can actually, to some extent, *induce* moodiness. Tensed stomach muscles can—again, to some extent—*induce* mental anxiety. This simple fact, obvious enough to anyone, is turned by yogis into a major key to the problem of self-development.

For, as physical tensions can induce, as well as reinforce, mental tensions, so physical relaxation can bring serenity to a worried mind. Ripples, after striking the shore of a pond, return toward their source. An effect, in its turn, is often found to affect its initial cause. If this first effect can be altered, the cause may be substantially altered also.

It is difficult to change one's mental outlooks. It is difficult even to view them objectively. The thoughts with which one would disperse his delusions are already poisoned by the very delusions he is trying to disperse!

To change oneself physically, however, in such a way as to influence the mind to adopt a similarly reformed outlook is a relatively simple undertaking. Harmonize the body, and it will be easier to harmonize the mind. This principle is fundamental to the science of hatha yoga. And it applies, in varying degrees of subtlety, to all levels of yoga teaching.

The breathing, for example, is affected by one's state of mind. Change the breathing, and one's mental state may be changed, too.

"But," you may ask, "how, specifically, can a bodily posture or a breathing exercise affect one's mental outlook?"

The connection between the body and the mind is the energy (*prana*) in the body. It is energy that transmits signals from the senses to the brain. It is energy that carries impulses from the brain to the body. When the flow of this energy is obstructed or set out of balance, there is a corresponding inharmony in both body and mind. The yoga postures are designed to promote and to harmonize the flow of energy in the body. The perceptive hatha yogi, understanding this truth, will endeavor to become conscious of his energy, and will use the postures and breathing exercises as a means primarily to developing this awareness. For *awareness is the first and most important stage towards gaining control.*

One of the most fascinating discoveries that the practicing yogi makes concerning his own psycho-physical nature is that the positive and negative currents, which we discussed earlier, have their literal counterpart in a directional flow of the energy in his body. When he thinks positively, there is an upward flow, literally, of this energy. When he thinks negatively, there is a downward flow. It is no accident that common parlance speaks of feeling "uplifted," "on top of the world," of feeling as though one's soul were "flying," when one feels happy.

Nor is it accidental that one speaks of feeling "downcast," "under the weather," "dragged down," "depressed," when he feels sad.

Yogis say that, in an uplifted state of awareness, the energy is literally concentrated in the upper part of the body. At such times, the very eyes tend to look upward, the corners of the mouth to turn up; everything about the body suggests an upliftment of this inner energy. But in a depressed state of mind, the energy becomes concentrated in the lower part of one's body: The eyes become downcast; the corners of the mouth turn downward; there is a sagging in the face, in the shoulders, in the arms; one's whole body suggests a sense of heaviness, of being earthbound.

It does not seem likely that heaven and hell are above us or below us in an objective sense, as tradition claims. But it is not difficult to demonstrate to oneself that heaven is up, and hell down, from a standpoint of one's own inner awareness.

An all-important purpose of the yoga postures, and indeed of all yoga practices, is to assist the direction of this inner energy toward the upper part of the body, especially toward the brain. Just as a calm, relaxed pose can help to induce a calm state of mind, even so, the simple process of changing the inner level of one's energy can have a tremendous effect on the quality of his awareness. By directing his energy upward, it becomes relatively easy for him to develop a positive mental outlook —to become kind, willing, energetic, and joyous.

For our virtues and vices are not really we, ourselves. They are reflections, only, of the plane of consciousness on which we live. As that plane changes, the traits of our personality change also.

Lest it be imagined that virtue can be developed by mechanics alone, it must be stressed that without an endeavor also to change the quality of one's thoughts, no deep-seated good can be achieved. Our thoughts are the *prime* cause of whatever harmony or inharmony we experience, not in the mind only, but in the body as well. To concentrate on soothing the effects while continuing to aggravate the initial cause would be like trying to placate a cat with milk while continuing to stand on its tail.

But if there is a sincere desire to improve one's state of mental awareness, then the yoga postures, the breathing exercises, and above all, the deliberate effort to harmonize and uplift one's inner energy, can be a tremendous aid to this worthwhile endeavor.

Basic Rules
for Yoga Practice

The yoga postures are very different from ordinary calisthenics. It is a mistake even to call these postures exercises, in the usual sense of the word. Their purpose is not to strengthen the muscles. They emphasize relaxation quite as much as they do tension. Unlike most physical exercise, they do not excite; rather, they eliminate excitement from the system.

With these thoughts in mind, the practitioner will understand that he has not "done" a posture once he has succeeded in assuming it. It is only at this point that he can begin truly to derive the benefits of that pose.

An important difference between these postures and calisthenics is that *in yoga practice one must never strain. Relax, never force yourself, into the prescribed positions.* Stretch only slightly, if at all, beyond the point of comfort. You will be astonished to see how many poses you can accomplish by progressively deeper relaxation.

Yogis illustrate their teaching of relaxation by the example of the cat. Observe this self-contained creature. It never uses more of its body at any given moment than it needs. Lift it up when it is resting, and observe how it hangs, limp, in your hands. Yet, so poised is it that, from a position of complete repose, it can leap to its feet in an instant, ready to defend itself against sudden danger.

The yogi, similarly, should act always from a center of poise and calmness, of mental and physical relaxation. When I first met the great yogi, Paramhansa Yogananda, he told me that, while sitting in a chair giving interviews, he was not even aware of his body below the chest. To be able so completely to relax the body when not using it, it is necessary first to be in full control of it, to be able at will to be fully conscious of every muscle.

The yoga postures, then, are not only a series of physical positions, but exercises in mental awareness. The yogi must be very deliberate in every movement. He must feel every muscle. Above all, he must try to become conscious of the energy as it directs the muscular movements. He must try to develop an awareness of his body as consisting primarily of energy.*

Between poses, he should calmly withdraw his energy from the periphery of his body; he should rest within himself. *Savasana*, the Corpse Pose, is particularly recommended for these peaceful interludes.

Diet plays an important, though not an essential, part in the life of the yogi. He should avoid foods that irritate or excite the system, and should eat mainly those which have a calming, harmonizing effect. Foods are rated by yogis according to whether they "heat" or "cool" the system. Fresh fruits, nuts, raw or lightly cooked vegetables, whole grains, milk and fresh milk products fall into the category of foods that have a cooling influence. Excessively spiced food, alcoholic beverages, too many carbohydrates, stimulants, and stale or devitalized foods are unnatural to the body, and are said to have a heating effect on it.

Meat, similarly, is considered unnatural to the human system. Swami Sri Yukteswar, the spiritual teacher of Paramhansa Yogananda, pointed out** that man's tooth structure is not that of a carnivorous animal, but rather that of a frugivorous, or fruit-eating, animal. His intestinal tract, too, measured from mouth to anus, is proportionately that of a frugivorous animal. Carnivores have intestinal tracts three to five times the length of their bodies; herbivores, 20 to 28 times that length. Frugivorous animals, including man, have intestinal tracts ten to twelve times the length of their bodies.

From an observation of natural sensory response, also, one can easily mark the pleasure of a carnivore at the

---

*No idle fancy, by the way. Science has proved that matter is energy.

**Sri Yukteswar, *The Holy Science*, Self-Realization Fellowship (Los Angeles, Calif.), pp. 39-45.

sight of raw meat and dripping blood. Man has the capacity to develop tastes outside his natural instinctual pattern, yet is it not usual for men to feel a repugnance for blood? As far as possible, the public sensibilities are protected from the massacre that goes on in a slaughter house. These places are so situated that sight, sound, and odor are kept as much as possible within their walls. Meat, when it is brought home, is carefully cooked and in other ways disguised.

No, meat is not man's *natural* food.

But who can deny the instinctive pleasure he feels at the sight and fragrance of fresh fruit? Unnatural living may have changed one's tastes and capacities from their instinctive norm, but self-analysis can hardly fail to confirm these observations at least to some extent.

Meat is an irritant to the human system. Yogis are not alone in claiming that it is the cause of many diseases in man; Western doctors, too, have been known to make such a claim. Nations of heavy meat-eaters are, as a general rule, more aggressive than nations whose primary diet is vegetarian. For a calm, inwardly centered, harmonious life, yogis recommend abstinence from meat. Other forms of protein are easily available, and are completely nourishing.

If a person is too strongly habituated to meat eating, however, or if he finds it inconvenient to give up meat altogether, he would do well at least to give up eating beef and pork, and to eat other meats less frequently.

The yogi is enjoined to practice moderation in everything. He should avoid eating too much, or too little. He should not sleep too much, nor too little. (More than seven hours' sleep in a night only drugs the nervous system.) He should be especially moderate in his sex life. Sexual over-indulgence causes a tremendous drain on a person's natural vitality. Continence, by contrast, provided it has the full consent of the mind, can be a tremendous factor in helping one to achieve full vigor, mentally and physically, and to attain deep spiritual insight.

Yoga practices help one to live in harmony with the forces of nature. The yoga practitioner should assist this harmonizing process by living as much as possible close to nature. He should get out into the countryside whenever he can, there to enjoy the sunshine, to breathe the fresh air. Yoga breathing exercises will help him to gain the greatest possible benefit from nature's free gift of oxygen.

In fact, the yoga postures should always, if possible, be practiced out-of-doors, or by an open window.

They should be practiced on an empty stomach, or at least three hours after eating. It is preferable that the body be warm when performing them. But don't practice immediately after strenuous activity. Don't practice so long, moreover, that the postures themselves result in over-exertion and fatigue.

Women should use caution if they wish to do yoga postures during the first day or two of the menstrual period. Pregnant women who want to continue their practice of the postures are advised to find one of the growing number of people who are specially trained in pre- and postnatal yoga.

The postures should not be practiced, save with the greatest of caution, when the body is unwell. Any posture that gives rise to a feeling of pain (other than muscular) in the chest, abdomen, or brain should be abandoned until the cause of pain has been ascertained. People with high blood pressure should avoid all but the most gentle poses.

One of the troubles that people have with the postures is the cramps that they get in the feet and in the legs. A deficiency in calcium is sometimes the cause, for which more calcium is the obvious cure. Cramps in the feet may be helped also by standing up, turning one foot back, and resting one's weight on the back side of the toes as much as possible, so as to bend the foot back further.

The duration of each posture must be increased *gradually*. People beginning these postures after middle age should be particularly careful to start slowly, with the easier poses, only bit by bit working up to the more difficult ones.

It is important, finally, to stress that persons who want to devote a great deal of time to these postures—to become, in short, hatha yogis, rather than persons who use hatha yoga as a means of achieving a more balanced, normal life—should practice them under a competent guide. Hatha yoga is not to be gone into *deeply* on one's own.

Special Note

The student has again and again been instructed in these pages to be aware of the energy in the body—of the flow of energy when the muscles are tensed, of the release of energy when the vertebrae are stretched. A method, not taught specifically in the science of hatha yoga, yet invaluable for a deeper understanding and mastery of this science, was discovered by Paramhansa Yogananda, the great yogi of modern India. His energization exercises may be learned from the organization that he founded: Self-Realization Fellowship, 3880 San Rafael Avenue, Los Angeles, California 90065.

2

Postures

The selection and sequence of these postures has been guided by the particular orientation of this book: the development of inner Self-awareness. Taking into account the fact that people have varied amounts of time for yoga practice, we have included in *Appendix C* routines of short and long duration.

Generally speaking, we have not followed the practice, common to most books on the subject, of cataloguing every muscle, tendon, gland, internal organ, bone, etc., that is supposed to be benefited by each pose. Readers who feel instructed by such a wealth of anatomical detail are recommended to the works of authors who share their fascination.

Nor have we included the long list of variations on each of these poses. This book is for people who want something simple, practical, and immediate. It is assumed that anyone who wants to become an expert on the subject will in any case go to a teacher, not to a book, for his instruction.

Standing Poses

*R*ight posture is vitally important to the yogi. A bent spine impairs the flow of energy. It also cramps the breath, making it almost impossible to breathe deeply.

Right posture, however, from a standpoint of yoga, is by no means the rigid stance of a soldier on parade. One must be relaxed even while standing straight. Indeed, until one can learn to keep his spine straight he will never know how to relax perfectly. Stand in such a way that you feel yourself centered in the spine, with the rest of your body suspended from the spine in much the same way as branches are suspended from the trunk of a tree. The chest should be somewhat (but not too much) out, the shoulders a little bit back, the head neither hanging forward nor drawn back too rigidly. If you stand perfectly straight, you will find that it takes very little strength to remain standing, only enough strength to maintain your balance.

The majority of the yoga postures relate to the development of awareness of the spine, either by stretching and irrigating the spine or by inducing a more centered consciousness.

Centeredness in the spine is important not only for spiritual awakening, but even in sports and in other daily human activities. I have found that when skiing, for example, that if I deliberately center my awareness in the spine, feeling all my movements to be radiating outward from that center, I can ski very much better. One who can remain consciously centered in the spine will always be poised, ready to meet any situation that arises.

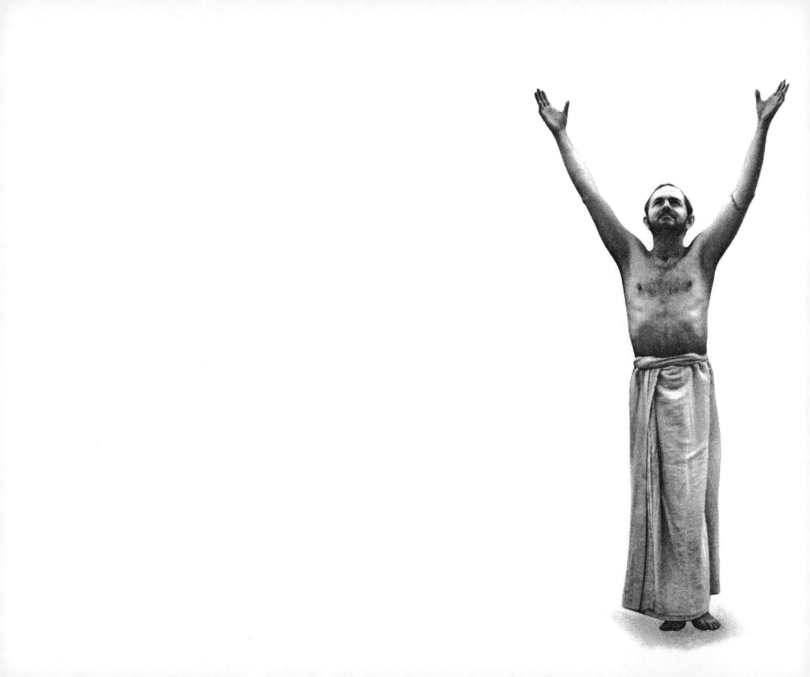

The Full Yogic Breath

Most people do not breathe as they should, owing to faulty posture, to wrong mental habits, and possibly even to the reluctance one feels in our modern environment to breathe air that is so generally impure. (Notice how often you tend to curb your natural breathing process when driving on the freeways or through a tunnel thick with exhaust fumes.)

The practice of deliberate, slow, deep breathing several times a day will gradually accustom your lungs to proper breathing habits. This does not mean that correct breathing must always be slow and deep. But this deep breathing practice will in time relax whatever muscular restrictions there are around the diaphragm, the sides, and the upper part of the chest, permitting the breath to flow freely and naturally at all times.

Diaphragmatic Breathing

To breathe properly, one should begin with the diaphragm, that membrane which separates the lungs from the visceral cavity. Air enters the lungs as they expand, creating a lower air pressure within the lungs than outside the body. The diaphragm works by a downward movement, which forces the stomach a little outward. If your stomach does not expand as you inhale, you are not breathing diaphragmatically.

Considering how important the diaphragm is to the breathing mechanism, it is alarming how few people breathe with it at all. Without proper breathing, true health is impossible. There are, of course, many causes of faulty diaphragmatic action. Poor posture is one—when a person stoops forward habitually, he cannot breathe diaphragmatically. Another cause is mental tension. Ulcers are a symptom of stomach tension—the result of intense mental anxiety. When the stomach is kept always tensed, diaphragmatic breathing is impossible. With diaphragmatic breathing, however, this tension may be gradually overcome. Proper breathing is, indeed, one of the most effective forms of psychotherapy.

Expanding the Ribs

The diaphragmatic expansion is only the first part of the full natural breathing process that has come to be called the Full Yogic Breath. The next stage is the outward movement of the floating ribs. People who hold themselves mentally too much inward from the threat of the world around them tend to become tensed physically around the sides of the ribs. People who breathe freely sideways tend to be courageous, expansive in their outlook. A deliberate effort to breathe outward sideways can help one to develop these wholesome attitudes.

Upper Chest

The third stage in a Full Yogic Breath is the one to which many people, women especially, limit themselves, though too few people breathe properly even here: the upper part of the chest. Development of the upper chest is associated with the capacity for feeling, for emotional expression. People whose chests are flat in the region above the breasts tend to be over-intellectual, emotionally repressed. Men are particularly at fault here. In the Full Yogic Breath the lungs are finally expanded to include this upper portion. By learning to breathe deeply here, one can help to enrich his capacity for emotional feeling.

One of the best ways to learn to breathe diaphragmatically is to lie flat on your back in *Savasana*, the Corpse Pose (page 55). Practice the whole technique of *Savasana* as explained, finally watching the navel rise and fall with the respiration. When the body is perfectly relaxed, as it is in sleep, diaphragmatic breathing becomes natural and effortless.

TECHNIQUE

A good technique for learning the Full Yogic Breath is to stand up and inhale as deeply as you can in a smooth, flowing motion. Again, begin with the diaphragm;

continue to the sides of the rib cage; lastly, fill the upper part of the lungs. Hold the breath several moments, then exhale slowly in reverse order.

○ It may help you to breathe more deeply if you begin by stooping forward, your arms hanging limply before you. Exhale.

○ Inhale first with the diaphragm and feel that the downward movement of this membrane, in pushing the stomach outward, is forcing your body gradually into an upright position. Feel also, as you inhale, that you are filling your lungs from the diaphragm, and not only your lungs but your whole body with air.

○ Straighten up slowly and bring your arms upward, your elbows out to the sides, your hands close to the body. Feel that you are stretching your rib cage outward, filling the middle part of your lungs.

○ Then, with a graceful movement, extend the arms upward and outward above your head, filling the upper part of your lungs, and imagine that the air is filling your arms all the way to the fingertips. Hold this position momentarily.

○ Then exhale slowly, lowering your arms and stooping forward again.

○ *Note:* With every inhalation, feel that you are drawing not only air, but strength, vitality, and joy into every body cell, from the toes all the way up to the crown of your head. With every exhalation, feel that you are expelling from your mental world all weakness and negativity.

○ With the last exhalation, lower your arms, but remain standing upright.

Note: A fuller discussion of the breath and principles of breathing appears in *Appendix A.*

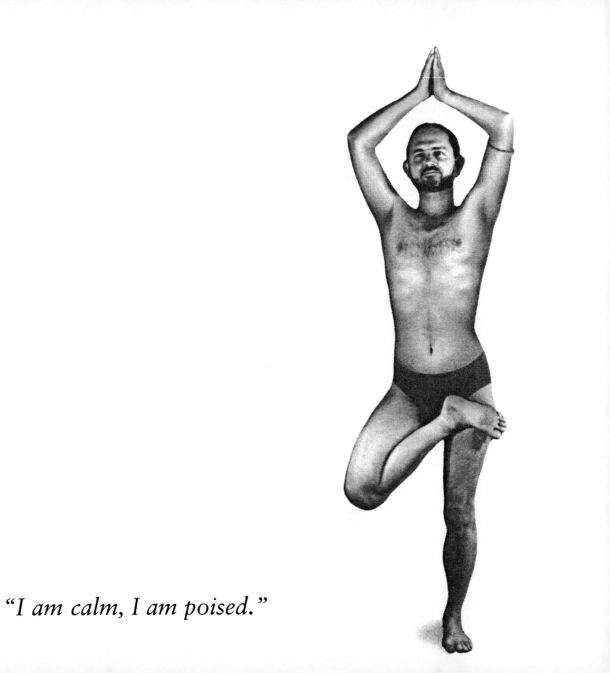

"I am calm, I am poised."

Vrikasana
THE TREE POSE

Vrikasana is an excellent posture with which to begin your daily practice of the postures. This *asana* will help you to feel more centered in yourself—an essential attitude for the successful performance of the ensuing poses. It will also help you to develop good posture.

TECHNIQUE

O Stand upright. Very slowly and calmly bring your right foot up and place it on the opposite thigh at the junction of the abdomen, pointing the knee downward. *Note:* If you find it difficult to bring your foot up as high as the junction of the thigh and abdomen, you may rest the instep against the inside of the opposite knee.

O Inhale and, standing as erect as possible, raise your arms slowly at the sides, keeping them straight, with palms upward, until the palms meet above the head.

O Mentally feel that there is a straight line extending upward through your spine to your joined hands and fingers. Feel that you are centered in this straight line. It is also helpful to focus on a point on the opposite wall or the floor. Relax your body as much as possible.

O Mentally affirm, "I am calm, I am poised."

O Hold this pose and concentrate on the inner feeling of centeredness for as long as you can do so comfortably.

O Exhale slowly, bringing your arms down slowly to the sides and lowering your foot to the floor.

O Repeat with the opposite leg.

"At the center of life's storms I stand serene."

Garudasana
THE TWISTED POSE

This pose is more difficult to describe than to practice! Its special benefit is psychological and spiritual, giving one a feeling of inner calmness and strength amidst the outer turmoil of life. *Garudasana* is a good pose for energizing the arms and legs.

TECHNIQUE

○ Stand on the left foot and bring the right leg in front of and around it as far as it will go.

○ Raise the left arm and bring the right arm simultaneously below and around the left, so that the elbows are interlocked and the palms of the hands are together. You may wish to raise your elbows up to feel a greater stretch across the upper back.

○ Stand straight, and feel your consciousness centered in the spine. Feel that, though life twists you outwardly in countless directions, inwardly you remain at peace, centered in your higher Self.

○ Affirm mentally, "At the center of life's storms I stand serene."

○ Stand on that leg as long as you find it comfortable to do so.

○ Repeat, standing on the right leg and alternating the position of the arms.

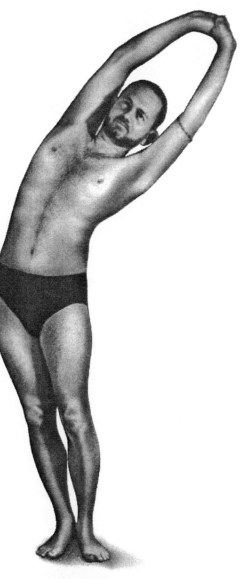

"Strength and courage fill my body cells."

Chandrasana
THE MOON POSE

Chandrasana will help make you more conscious of the spine, a vital necessity in more advanced poses.

TECHNIQUE

○ Stand with your feet together, with the weight on the balls of the feet. Be conscious now of your spine—imagine that a rising current of energy in the spine is extending upward beyond the shoulders.

○ Inhale slowly and bring your arms out to the sides, palms upward, and straight up above your head. As your hands meet, lock your thumbs together with your palms facing forward, stretch upward, and rise up on your toes.

○ Now exhale, shifting the right hip to the right, and extend the stretch of the upper body to the left. Remain slightly up on your toes. Try not to twist the body, but keep it flat, as though you were bending between two panes of glass.

○ Be aware of the upward movement of energy in your body, as if it were the energy itself that is stretching your body and extending the stretch to the left.

○ Affirm mentally, "Strength and courage fill my body cells."

○ Hold this pose for approximately 30 seconds, breathing naturally when you need to.

○ Inhale, returning to the upright position. Stretch upward again.

○ Exhale and bring your arms slowly down to your sides, settling back onto your heels.

○ Repeat *Chandrasana* in the opposite direction.

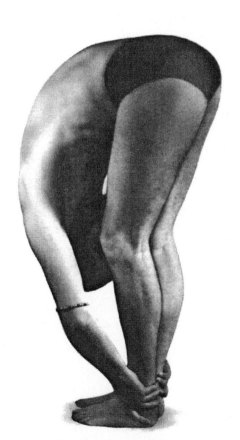

"What in this world can hold me?"

Padahastasana

THE JACKKNIFE POSE — *moving into* THE BACKWARD BEND

The yogi is taught, as an exercise in mental freedom, to meditate on vast space. Normally, such spatial awareness is obstructed by one's sense of physical heaviness. In *Padahastasana*, this natural sense of gravity is disoriented by the half-upward, half-downward position of the body. The mind is more easily freed from its gravitational bondage.

It is somewhat more difficult to keep the legs straight in this position than in the sitting stretches, where the pressure of the floor may be used to good advantage. Here there is no such pressure to suggest straightness to the legs. From a standpoint, then, of the stretch of the upper body, this pose is easier than the sitting stretches, but from a standpoint of keeping the legs straight, it is more difficult.

Padahastasana exercises a beneficial pressure on the abdomen. It helps to stretch the spine in a slightly different manner from the sitting stretches, inasmuch as here the entire weight of the upper body is brought into play.

TECHNIQUE

○ Stand up straight.

○ Inhale deeply, drawing the arms up over the head and stretching the spine. Now exhale and bend forward from the hips, keeping a straight back. Feel as though you are reaching out for the opposite wall.

○ Relax fully forward, keeping the weight over the balls of the feet, and grasp the ankles. Breathe normally in this position. *Note:* You may, if you prefer, grasp the toes in a more complete forward stretch.

○ While in this posture, drop your head and relax at the base of the spine. Keep the legs as straight as possible. *Note:* You will find that the more you relax at the base of the spine, the more easily you will be able to bend forward.

○ Affirm mentally, "What in this world can hold me?"

○ Hold the position for about ten seconds to start with, gradually increasing the time with practice to about one minute.

○ Inhale and return slowly to an upright position by uncurling the back. Feel as though you are placing one vertebra on top of the next as you move up.

Follow the Jackknife Pose with the Backward Bend:

○ Standing upright, put one foot in front of the other.

○ Inhale and raise your hands forward and upward, palms turned up, until you can join your palms together above the head. Stretch upward and backward.

○ Feel the triumphant freedom that is suggested by this position. Feel your energy and consciousness being swept upward to the sky.

○ Affirm mentally, "I am free! I am free!"

○ Repeat, placing the other foot forward.

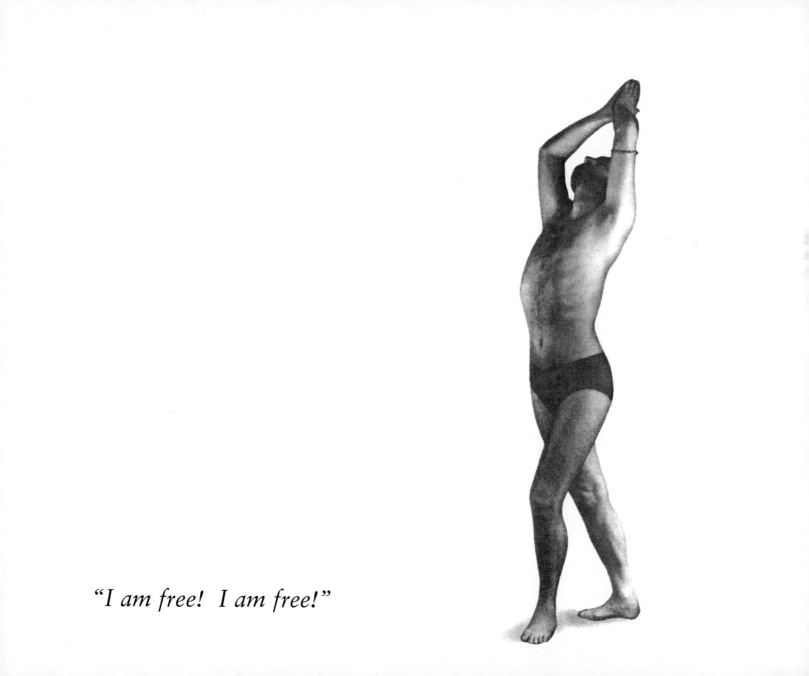

"*I am free! I am free!*"

*"Energy and joy flood my body cells!
Joy descends to me!"*

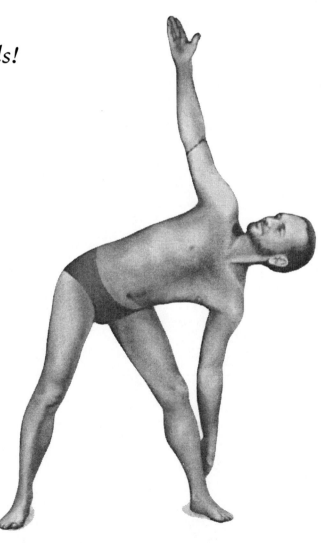

Trikonasana
THE TRIANGLE POSE

In *Chandrasana*, the Moon Pose, the stretch is completely to the side. In the Triangle Pose there is a slight forward angle to the stoop, which provides a different kind of stretch to the back.

TECHNIQUE

O Stand with feet spread apart, at least to shoulder width.

O Inhale, lifting the arms outward to the sides, palms upward, and stretch back slightly.

O Now exhale slowly, bending over and slightly forward to the left until your left hand touches the left foot. Extend the right arm upward above your head, turning your head to look up at the outstretched fingers.

O Affirm mentally, "Energy and joy flood my body cells! Joy descends to me!"

O Hold the pose as long as you find it comfortable—approximately 30 seconds for most people.

O Inhale and return slowly to a standing position. Stretch your arms out sidewise, palms upward, then slowly exhale as you allow your arms to come down to your sides again.

O Repeat the same movements to the right.

"My body is no burden; it is light as air."

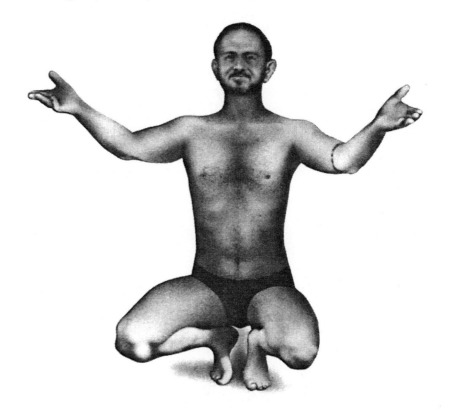

Utkatasana
THE CHAIR POSE

The Chair Pose is valuable psychologically. It suggests to the mind a sense of lightness and vitality, a freedom from bondage to the heavy, downward pull of Earth.

Utkatasana also tones the leg muscles and helps (in the second phase) to relieve tired feet.

TECHNIQUE

○ Stand upright. Inhale, raising your arms straight out in front of you, palms up, and rise up simultaneously on your toes as you raise your arms.

○ Then crouch down part way, as if you were sitting down but were so light that you needed nothing but air to rest upon.

○ Affirm mentally, "My body is no burden; it is light as air."

○ For the second phase of this posture, squat down all the way, remaining on your toes. In this position, place your hands on your hips.

○ When you are ready to come up again, sweep your arms forward and upward, with the palms turned up. Inhale as you come up and raise your arms in a graceful sweeping motion over your head, backward, and down as you settle back onto the heels, exhaling.

Relaxation Poses

*I*t is impossible to develop true Self-awareness without first learning how to relax. Energy that is bound cannot soar to divine heights. The science of yoga might even be defined as a process of progressive relaxation: first, from outer attachments; then from attachment to body, to thoughts, to personality, to ego—until one finds himself at last in the stream of infinite life.

To withdraw one's mind from worldly attachment is a prerequisite to deeper relaxation. But this is no easy task. The mind functions on many levels of which man is only dimly aware. Even when the mind tries consciously to withdraw from outward distractions, subconscious habit patterns may continue to direct the energy on its customary outward course, tensing the body, putting "knots" in the nerves, imprisoning the energy in the muscles and nerve channels.

Desire for outward activity causes tension. This tension is especially noticeable in the legs and arms. The tendons above the feet, the front part of the calves and thighs, contract automatically with the impulse to be "up and doing." The arms, the front part of the armpits, the fingers (especially the little fingers and the thumbs and forefingers, where important nerves have their endings)—here, too, tension reflects any inner need to "swing" into action.

The desire for activity originates in the mind, but, like the steady increase of sound that occurs in "feedback" between a loudspeaker and a microphone, tension augments that initial desire. A relaxed body makes it much easier to arrest this steady build-up, to withdraw the energy and thereby to calm the mind. Most of the difficulty people experience in meditation stems from physical tension. When a person is completely relaxed, it is easy to sit still even for hours at a time.

How to relax physically? Paramhansa Yogananda explained the matter more lucidly than any other recent writer. He taught that, for physical relaxation, one must first become conscious of existing tension. To develop this consciousness, first, increase that tension deliberately. Tense the whole body. When fully conscious of this tension, release it completely; become altogether limp and motionless. *

We begin relaxation by stretching and tensing the extremities of the body—those parts, especially, which respond to the impulse for physical activity.

---

* There are psychological corollaries to this principle. Suffering, for example, must be completely accepted before it can be overcome and forgotten.

"I am the master;
   all body energies are at my command!"

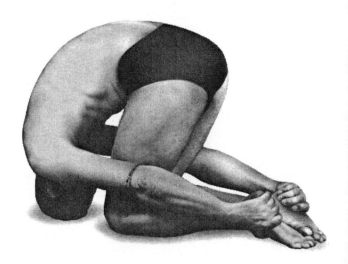

Sasamgasana
THE HARE POSE

When the mind is eager to swing into activity, messages are sent to those parts of the body which make outward activity possible. Tensions appear in the shoulders (especially in the front part of the armpits), between the shoulder blades, and in the arms. *Sasamgasana*, by stretching and then relaxing these parts, helps to free the mind of their suggestion, through feedback, that one should be continuously busy doing things.

The Hare Pose is excellent for relaxing these body parts. If, in doing this pose, you are able to squat down completely on your calves, the gentle pressure of the weight on your legs, feet, and abdomen will also help to relieve fatigue in the lower body.

The gentle inversion of the body will bring blood to your brain and benefit the sinuses. Because it is refreshing to the brain, *Sasamgasana* helps to banish mental fatigue.

Sasamgasana is a good pose to practice before meditation.

TECHNIQUE

○ Sit in *Vajrasana*, the Firm Pose (page 115). *Note:* If you cannot sit down all the way, it won't matter for the purposes of this pose.

○ Exhale and bend slowly forward, leading with your chin and keeping a flat back, until your head touches the floor in front of you, close to your knees. Put your hands backward and down by your sides.

○ Rest in that position, breathing normally, for 30 seconds to one minute.

○ Now draw the forehead up closer to your knees and grasp your heels firmly with your hands in such a way that the fingers are curled inward, not outward, upon the heels.

○ Raise the buttocks, bringing the weight of the upper body onto the top of the head, until your arms are stretched straight and held taut by the grip of the hands on the heels.

○ You should feel a stretch in the shoulders, between the shoulder blades, in the front part of the armpits, and down the arms to the fingers. *Note:* If you do not feel a pull in these parts (if, for instance, your arms are too long to be stretched straight in this position) turn the elbows one way or another until you do feel an actual pull.

○ Be very conscious of this stretch, affirming mentally, "I am the master; all body energies are at my command!"

○ Relax now with your forehead on the floor; inhale and slowly return to *Vajrasana* again, keeping your back flat.

○ You may want to rest in *Savasana*, the Corpse Pose (page 55), and feel the energy withdrawing from your hands, arms, and shoulders to the spine.

*"I am the master;
all body energies are at my command!"*

"Energetic movement or unmoving peace:
The choice is mine alone! The choice is mine!"

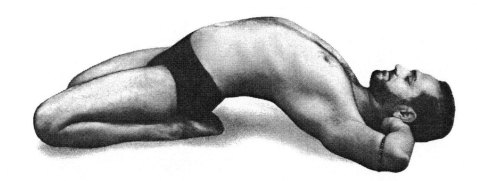

Supta-Vajrasana
THE SUPINE FIRM POSE

The lower part of the body tends to become tensed as a result of the mind's inclination to be "up and doing." Every such impulse from the mind, no matter how tentative, sends corresponding impulses to the thighs, the skin muscles, the feet. Such tensions often linger even after the mind has moved on to other thoughts. Repeated impulses create a gradual build-up of tension in those parts to the point where, like unruly children, they cry for attention, often drowning out all wishes to the contrary in the conscious mind. The meditating devotee may desire to sit still, lost in inner peace, but tensions in the legs keep shouting at him with vociferous silence to be "up and doing," until at last in despair, he leaves his meditation.

Supta-Vajrasana is a marvelous pose for relaxing the parts of the legs that have been described and thus for preparing the body for deep meditation.

In addition to the benefits mentioned above, this pose is excellent for the stomach and for correcting postural defects.

The Camel Pose, offered on page 51 as an alternate to *Supta-Vajrasana*, is excellent for the pelvis and for toning the muscles in the stomach and back.

TECHNIQUE

○ To assume this position, sit in *Vajrasana*, the Firm Pose (page 115).

○ Lean backward slowly, using the hands and elbows for support, until the top of your head touches the floor behind you. *Note:* To go more fully into this position it is important that you be relaxed. If, therefore, this pose is too difficult for you, it would be helpful to use a low box or cushion on which to rest your shoulders, instead of straining to hold yourself bent back as far as possible. In whatever position you relax, whether resting on the top of your head or on a low box, you will find over a period of 30 seconds or so that you can go back further still. By progressive relaxation you may find, to your surprise, that the full supine position is not so difficult after all.

○ To assume the full position, raise your arms and clasp the hands beneath the head.

○ Slowly come down, *without raising your knees*, until your shoulders rest on the floor. The longer you hold this position, the more you will be surprised at how comfortable it can be! The knees should be as nearly together as possible.

○ In this position, affirm mentally, "Energetic movement or unmoving peace: The choice is mine alone! The choice is mine!"

○ When coming out of *Supta-Vajrasana*, do not sit up again, but roll over onto one hip, extend your legs slowly, and settle back comfortably into *Savasana*, the Corpse Pose (page 55). Resting in this position, repeat the affirmation and feel that you are sinking peacefully into the center of your being.

alternate position: THE CAMEL POSE

TECHNIQUE

○ Sit in *Vajrasana*.

○ Come up on your knees so that you are kneeling straight, as if praying in the Western tradition.

○ Bend backward at the waist until you can rest your hands on your heels.

○ Drop the head back and thrust the hips forward so as to form an arch between the head and the knees.

○ Hold this position not more than 15 seconds to start with, gradually increasing to a maximum of one minute.

○ Sit back slowly in *Vajrasana*.

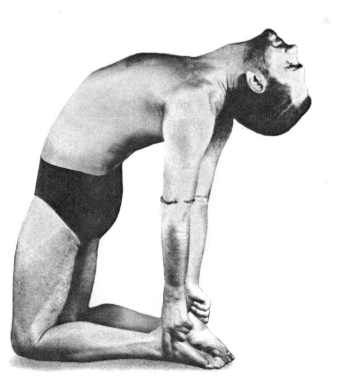

My soul floats on waves of cosmic light."

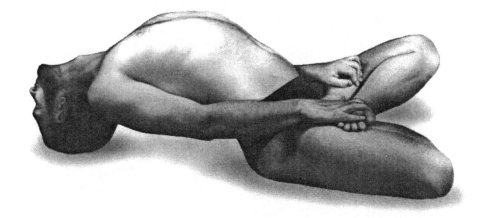

Matsyasana
THE FISH POSE

The Fish Pose is so called because in it one is supposed to be able to float comfortably in water. The reason for floating in water in conjunction with yoga practice is the mental freedom that this practice gives. One should feel that he is floating on waves of cosmic light, completely submissive to the ebb and flow of divine grace.

Rajarsi Janakananda (James J. Lynn), Paramhansa Yogananda's most advanced disciple in the West, used to practice *Matsyasana* while floating in the ocean at Encinitas, California. Rising and falling gently with the ocean waves, he soon found himself floating in *samadhi* on waves of cosmic consciousness.

Matsyasana is excellent as a follow-up to the forward bends, especially *Halasana*, the Plow Pose, and *Sarvangasana*, the Shoulderstand. It helps to overcome a stiff neck resulting from bending forward over a desk, or from sewing or reading.

Matsyasana also helps to draw energy upward to the spiritual eye.

TECHNIQUE

○ Sit in *Padmasana*, the Lotus Pose (page 123). If you cannot assume the full Lotus Pose, some of the benefits of *Matsyasana* may be achieved by simply sitting cross-legged and arching backward until your head touches the floor behind you.

○ Grasp the feet and lie back, keeping the knees down, until your head touches the floor behind you. (A variation of this pose is to join your hands under your head, bringing the shoulders down to the floor.)

○ *Matsyasana* may be held as long as one wishes.

○ While practicing either variation of this pose, affirm, "My soul floats on waves of cosmic light."

"Bones, muscles, movement I surrender now;
anxiety, elation and depression, churning thoughts—
all these I give into the hands of peace."

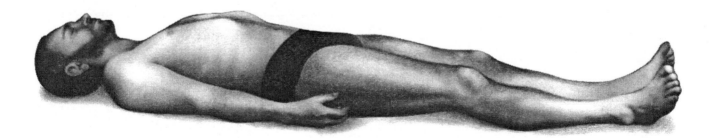

Savasana
THE CORPSE POSE

I have already pointed out the importance of being aware enough of one's body to relax it, and of relaxing into every pose instead of forcing oneself into them. It is time now to learn the supreme relaxation pose, *Savasana.*

On the surface, this would seem to be the simplest of all the poses to assume. In fact, however, because relaxation itself is so difficult, perfection in *Savasana* is rarely attained.

I have said that awareness is the necessary precursor of relaxation. There are many parts of the body that are tense without our conscious knowledge. How are we to become enough aware of them to relax them? The answer is, by increasing the tension throughout the body. Often it happens on a psychological level that we overcome our faults only when they have become so exaggerated as to be obvious to us. The same is true with physical tension. The best way to induce preliminary relaxation in the body is first to inhale, tense the whole body (equalizing the flow of tension throughout the body), then throw the breath out and relax the entire body at once. (This is the method taught by Paramhansa Yogananda for achieving preliminary overall relaxation.)

Savasana may be practiced more briefly between the other postures, until the heartbeat and the breathing have returned to normal. At the end of one's posture session, however, one should go into deep relaxation in *Savasana* for at least five or ten minutes, or until you have felt the deeper rejuvenating effects of total relaxation.

Relaxation may be particularized after each posture. If you have been stretching a particular part of the body (as, for example, the lower back in *Paschimotanasana,* the Posterior Stretching Pose), while doing *Savasana* after it concentrate especially upon the relaxation of the lower back, rather than on the relaxation of the whole body.

In addition to bringing supreme relaxation, *Savasana* helps in the development of receptivity, so important to yogic practice; rejuvenates the body cells; and aids in mental and physical healing.

TECHNIQUE

O Lie flat on your back, your legs outstretched, your hands, palms upward, at your sides. *Note:* Some people find they can relax better with the palms turned downward. If such is your case, follow the demands of your physical structure. Palms upward is the ideal position, however, as it induces a feeling of surrender, of trust; it conduces to mental as well as to physical relaxation.

O Inhale deeply, a short breath followed by a long one. Exhale similarly, short and long. Repeat two or three times.

O Then inhale, tense the whole body (equalizing the flow of tension throughout the body), throw the breath out and relax the entire body at once. Repeat two or three times.

O After this preliminary relaxation, lie very still. Be aware of your breath, if you like. You may watch it in the nostrils or simply be mentally aware of the rhythmic rise and fall of your navel. As your calmness deepens, feel your consciousness becoming centered increasingly at the point between the eyebrows.

O Now, strive for *deep* relaxation. Think of the body as surrounded by space—space in all directions spreading out to infinity.

O Think of your feet and visualize this space gradually seeping through the pores of the skin into your feet, until your feet become space. Visualize the space as gradually coming up into the calves, thighs, hips, the abdomen and stomach, the hands, forearms, upper arms, shoulders, chest, the back of the neck, sides of the neck, the throat, jaw, tongue, lips, cheeks, eyes, and brain.

○ In feeling space in your brain, release from your mind all regrets about the past, all worries about the future. Rest in the infinite ocean of the eternal Present. The objects of endless human concern no longer exist. There is nothing in all eternity but the Right Here, the Right Now.

○ Affirm mentally, "Bones, muscles, movement I surrender now; anxiety, elation and depression, churning thoughts—all these I give into the hands of peace."

Spinal Stretches

*N*ow, with the spinal limbering postures, we proceed to a deeper level in our development of Self-awareness. This third set of postures stretches the vertebrae. It opens subtle nerve channels, making possible the free movement of energy in the spine. This movement is important, not only physically, but mentally and spiritually as well. Physically, a free flow of energy in the spine floods the body with strength and vitality.

Mentally and spiritually, freeing the nerve channels of physical obstructions makes it easier to direct the energy upward, to the higher centers and to the brain.

"I am safe, I am sound.
All good things come to me; they give me peace!"

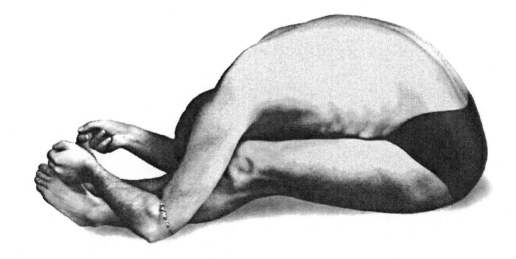

Paschimotanasana
THE POSTERIOR STRETCHING POSE

Modern day insecurity creates in man many tensions. Among these is a chronic tightness behind the knees, the result of a mental shrinking away from expected dangers and difficulties. Releasing the tension behind the knees can help, indirectly, to overcome this sense of insecurity. Coupled with mental affirmation, especially while resting in *Savasana*, the Corpse Pose (page 55), after the practice, the effect can be considerable.

It might be well, therefore, to practice this posture twice, the first time giving special attention to the knees, the second to the lower spine. During the rest period following the first practice, concentrate on the feeling of release in the legs behind the knees and affirm, "I am safe, I am sound. All good things come to me; they give me peace!" After the second practice, feel the surge of joy and vitality rising from your lower spine toward the brain.

Because of its stretching action on the tendons in the legs, *Paschimotanasana* is also an excellent limbering exercise to practice before attempting the more difficult of the sitting postures. The main stretch is, as the name of the posture implies, in the lower part of the back, but there also is a stretch in the tendons behind the knees—a secondary but very real purpose of the exercise. The stretch in the lower back releases energy to flow freely to and from that area of the spine. The stretch behind the knees, too, is useful in more ways than physical—it helps to release certain deep-seated psychological tensions.

Paschimotanasana helps to tone up the nervous system. It improves the functioning of the abdominal and pelvic organs and is excellent generally for digestion. *Note:* This posture is also used for transmuting sexual energy. In this context it is called *Brahmacharyasana*.

TECHNIQUE

○ Sit on the floor with your legs stretched out in front of you.

○ Inhale, then exhale slowly and stretch forward

slowly from the hips. Don't pull your body, but feel that you are offering yourself into the posture.

O Relax forward, keeping your legs flat on the floor, until your fingers can grasp the big toe of each foot, your elbows touch the floor, and your whole upper body can rest on the thighs, with your head on your knees or a little below them. The proper way, if you can do it, is to grasp the big toe with the thumb, forefinger, and middle finger of each hand, just as if you were grasping an upright post. *Note:* Stretch forward only as far as you can comfortably. This is not an easy pose to assume, particularly for older people. If you cannot reach your feet, then grasp your ankles or knees or whatever you can to steady your upper body.

O Be aware of the tension under the knees and at the base of the spine that is preventing you from going farther forward. Think space at these points of tension, and you will notice, surprisingly, that after a few moments you will be able to bend farther forward without any strain. Repeat this process, and over a minute or two you will see that you have bent forward much farther than you may have thought possible.

O Affirm mentally, "I am safe, I am sound. All good things come to me; they give me peace!"

O Gradually lie back and rest in *Savasana*, the Corpse Pose, for a minute or two.

O *Note:* The more difficult you find this position, the more vital your need for it. Beginners should not hold this pose more than 15 to 30 seconds. When you can do so comfortably, hold the pose up to three minutes.

"I am safe, I am sound.
All good things come to me; they give me peace!"

"Left and right
and all around—
life's harmonies are mine."

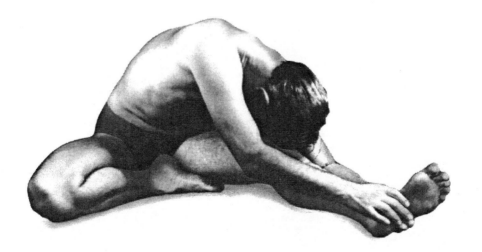

Janushirasana
THE HEAD-TO-THE-KNEE POSE

Janushirasana augments the benefits that are to be derived from *Paschimotanasana*, the Posterior Stretching Pose. It also helps to tone up the nervous system, improves the functioning of the abdominal and pelvic organs, and is excellent generally for digestion. Because of its stretching action on the tendons in the legs, it also is an excellent limbering exercise to practice before attempting the more difficult of the sitting postures.

TECHNIQUE

○ Sit on the floor, extending your legs outward in front of you, separating them into as wide an angle as is comfortable for you.

○ Bring the right foot in and place it in the crotch.

○ Inhale, raising the hands gracefully up the sides of the chest as if to draw the awareness into and up the spine. Then exhale slowly, turning to face the outstretched left leg and bending forward over it. As you bend forward, inwardly feel that you are surrendering yourself and releasing both psychological and physical tensions.

○ Grasp the foot with your hands and bring the head slowly forward until the forehead rests upon the knee. *Note:* If you cannot grasp your foot, then grasp ankle or calf to give your upper body the support it needs to relax properly. If you cannot touch your head to your knee, do not bring your knee up to touch your head (like Mohammed, who said that if the mountain would not come to him, he would go to the mountain!). Keep the outstretched leg straight and bring your head as far down to it as it will *comfortably* go. (This is a head-to-the-knee pose, not a knee-to-the-head pose!)

○ With the forward bends, it helps to use the breath to relax into the pose. With each inhalation, feel the vertebrae stretching, and with each exhalation feel the spine relaxing forward. You will find by progressive relaxation that you can bend farther and farther forward, until you have mastered the pose.

O Affirm mentally, "Left and right and all around—life's harmonies are mine."

O Hold the pose only a few seconds to begin with, increasing the time gradually to one or two minutes as it becomes comfortable to you.

O Return to a comfortable cross-legged pose and sit for a moment.

O Repeat, with the other leg outstretched.

*"Left and right
and all around—
life's harmonies are mine."*

"New life, new consciousness flow freely.
See: They flood my brain!"

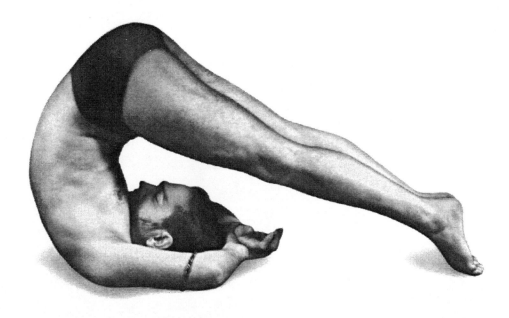

Halasana
THE PLOW POSE

This pose is one of the most important in hatha yoga. Many parts of the body are benefitted by it. Gratifyingly, it is also not too difficult to assume, but proceed gently just the same. Up to now, the energy has been released to flow through the lower part of your spine. It must now be given free passage through the upper spine. *Halasana* helps to accomplish this important end.

Halasana itself is good for the abdominal muscles and for the posture, besides its prime purpose of releasing the energy to flow freely in the upper spine. The Third and Fourth Phases of this pose are beneficial not only for stretching the upper spine and the neck, but also for the gentle stimulation they give the thyroid gland when the chest is pressed hard against the chin.

Holding the legs at a 45-degree angle helps to tone the muscles of the thighs and abdomen. This pose also brings blood into the brain.

In all of the yoga postures one should be deeply aware of every body movement, of every muscle that is brought into play. In *Halasana*, because so many parts of the body are involved, it is especially important to keep this principle of awareness in mind. Breathe normally in all phases of the pose.

TECHNIQUE

○ Lie flat on your back with arms down at your sides, palms down. Relax.

○ Inhale, press the small of the back to the floor, and raise both legs simultaneously, keeping them straight, to an angle of approximately 45 degrees from the floor. Be aware of the various muscles involved in the action.

○ Hold this position briefly, feeling the tension in the thighs and abdomen.

○ Now raise the legs slowly until they are perpendicular to the floor. Hold them there momentarily, feeling the pressure of the entire back against the floor.

○ Then, starting with the lower spine, release this pressure bit by bit as you continue to bring your legs up over your head until they are in a position parallel to the floor.

○ Hold this position a few moments, deeply relaxing your spine to prevent any strain when you assume *Halasana* itself. Then come down into the First Phase of the Plow Pose.

○ *First Phase:* Bring the feet down to the floor as close to your head as is comfortable. Feel the stretch in the lower and middle back. The knees should eventually be right above the eyes, with the legs kept straight. *Note:* Those who find the stretch initially to be more than they can manage may lower their feet to a chair or some cushions.

○ *Second Phase:* When you feel relaxed in the First Phase, move the feet back somewhat farther and feel the stretch extending up into the middle and upper back. Hold this position, too, until you feel relaxed in it.

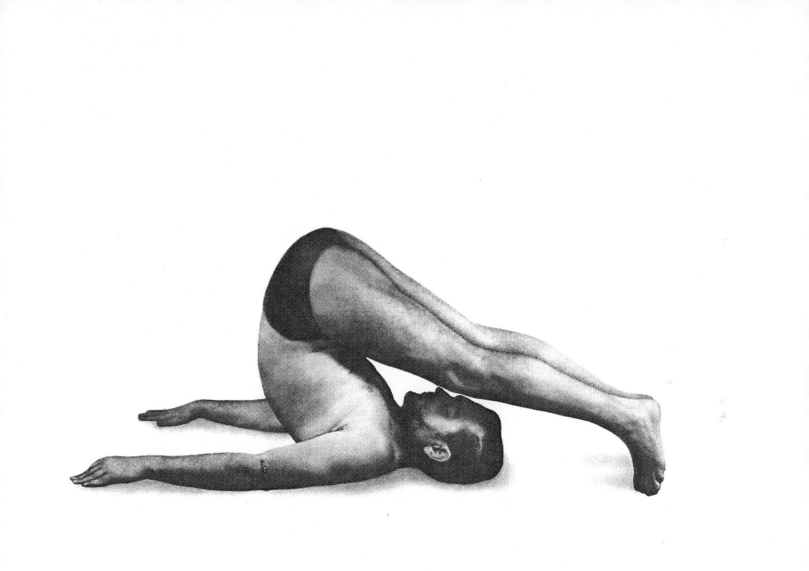

○ *Third Phase:* Then go back as far as you can and feel the stretch extending up into the upper back and lower neck.

○ *Fourth Phase:* Finally, bring your arms up above your head, and you will find that you can extend even farther back, stretching the upper vertebrae in the neck. The chin should be firmly pressed into the chest.

○ While in the Fourth Phase, affirm mentally, "New life, new consciousness flow freely. See: They flood my brain!"

○ Hold the pose for 30 seconds to begin with—up to two minutes with practice—then return slowly, vertebra by vertebra, back through the different phases to the supine position and rest awhile, lying flat on the floor. *Note:* You may benefit more from this posture if you repeat it several times, though in our experience deep relaxation makes more than one practice unnecessary. In any case, beginners should limit themselves to two or three attempts.

"New life, new consciousness flow freely.
See: They flood my brain!"

*"My boat of life
floats lightly on tides of peace."*

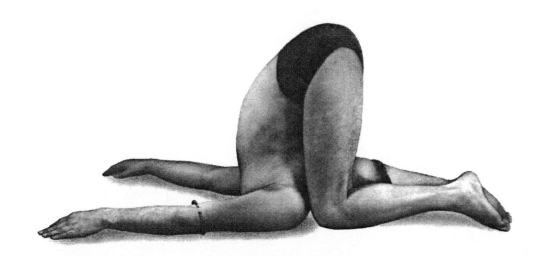

Karnapirasana
THE EAR-CLOSING POSE

Karnapirasana, once you can assume it comfortably, is surprisingly restful to the brain, as well as to the body. It is an excellent pose for tired businessmen after a hard day's work at the office!

TECHNIQUE

O Go into *Halasana*, the Plow Pose (page 69).

O Simply drop your knees down to the floor, pressing them against the shoulders and closing the ears. You may clasp the arms around the thighs, holding onto the right forearm with the left hand and left forearm with the right hand; or simply extend the arms over the head as in *Halasana*.

O One may affirm mentally while holding this position, "My boat of life floats lightly on tides of peace."

O Hold this position as long as you like, but not longer than one minute.

"*I rise determinedly to meet all obstacles.*"
Or: "*I rise joyfully to meet each new opportunity.*"

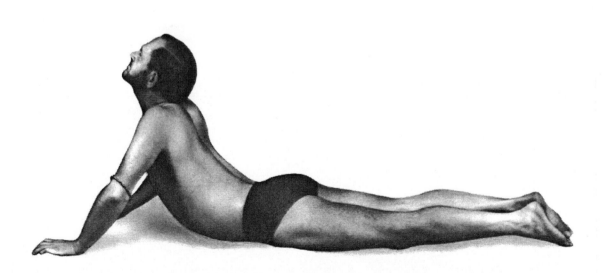

Bhujangasana
THE COBRA POSE

Forward-stretching poses should always be followed by others that stretch backward. It is, indeed, in this backward stretch that one becomes most conscious of the benefits that he has derived from the preceding stretches. It would seem, at least from our experience, that the forward-stretching poses open the nerve channels in the spine, but that the backward-stretching ones help to pour energy through those opened channels.

The reader who has any knowledge of the yoga postures will probably be familiar with the Cobra Pose. This pose is easy to assume; its benefits are great.

The psychological and spiritual benefits are most important. Psychologically the Cobra Pose increases one's strength to overcome obstacles. Spiritually it increases awareness of, and hence control over, the subtle energy in the spine.

The Cobra Pose stretches and straightens the upper spine and is relaxing to the spine in general. It also refreshes the brain. It strengthens the back and buttock muscles and exerts a gentle, beneficial pressure on the visceral organs. It helps one particularly to overcome flatulence after meals. *A word of caution:* People with enlarged liver or spleen ought not to practice this exercise or its sequel, *Dhanurasana*, the Bow Pose.

TECHNIQUE

○ Lie face downward with the palms flat against the floor at about shoulder level, elbows close to the body, and forehead resting on the floor.

○ Without using the arms, slowly raise the forehead, feeling the tension at the back of the neck, and graze the face lightly against the floor as you draw the head slowly farther and farther back until the shoulders are lifted off the ground. Continue to draw the back slowly upward until you can raise it no farther by its own strength. Concentrate not on the tension itself, but on the gathering of energy in the spine.

○ Then, with the arms, push yourself upward as far as your body will bend, *without raising your navel from the floor*. As you raise your back slowly, feel the gradual course of energy downward from the head through the spine with the tensing of each successive portion of the neck and back.

○ After attaining the final position, relax; you will find that you can bend farther still. Relax between the shoulder blades and push forward with the breastbone.

○ Visualize yourself as rising bravely to meet the challenge of all obstacles in your life. Affirm mentally, "I rise determinedly to meet all obstacles," or, "I rise joyfully to meet each new opportunity."

○ After five or ten seconds in the final position (as much as three minutes for adepts), return slowly to the supine position, reversing the sequence of tension and feeling the energy flow back up the spine to the brain.

○ *Note:* Repeat this posture, if you like, three to seven times, resting briefly between each practice. Beginners may breathe naturally, but after proficiency is attained one should inhale slowly while bending upward, and exhale slowly while returning to the first position.

"I rise determinedly to meet all obstacles."
Or: *"I rise joyfully to meet each new opportunity."*

"I recall my scattered forces
 to recharge my spine."

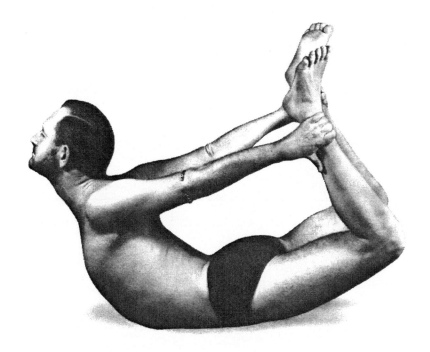

Dhanurasana
THE BOW POSE

This pose completes what *Bhujangasana*, the Cobra Pose, began. The Cobra Pose bends the upper spine backward. *Dhanurasana* bends the middle and lower spine. You will find your awareness of energy increasing if you hold the pose slightly beyond the point of comfort, though never, of course, to the point of pain. Concentrate on your feeling in the spine, not in the tensed muscles, and you will discover you can hold this pose long past what you might consider your limit of "strength."

The benefits of *Dhanurasana* are much the same as those for *Bhujangasana*. Physically, the gentle pressure of this pose upon the abdomen helps to stimulate the internal organs and to reduce flatulence. Psychologically, the Bow Pose increases one's strength to overcome obstacles. More important still are the spiritual benefits: *Dhanurasana* is a wonderful pose for awakening and increasing your awareness of, and hence control over, the subtle energy in the spine. A *word of caution:* People with enlarged liver or spleen ought not to practice this position or *Bhujangasana*.

TECHNIQUE

○ Lie face downward. Bend your legs at the knee and, reaching back with the hands, firmly grasp ankles or feet. Lie in this position with your forehead on the floor.

○ Inhale and, with the strength of your legs, pull your feet away from the body, forcing your chest and knees up off the floor until your weight rests solely on the abdomen. Keep the knees as close together as possible. Discomfort from lower back compression may be avoided by pushing the lower abdomen (the pelvic girdle) firmly to the floor and stretching and elongating the upper spine. *Note:* Breathe normally in this position. Be keenly aware of the bend in the lower spine. Feel the awakening of the energy there, and the drawing of energy to the lower spine from the legs.

○ Affirm mentally, "I recall my scattered forces to recharge my spine." (Or visualize yourself floating cheerfully over the crests of all difficulties and affirm mentally, "Each wave of trials can only raise me to new heights.")

○ Hold this pose as long as you can do so comfortably. Then return slowly to a prone position. *Note:* You may repeat this posture two or three times if you like, with short rests in between.

"I recall my scattered forces
to recharge my spine."

"I am awake!
Energetic!
Enthusiastic!"

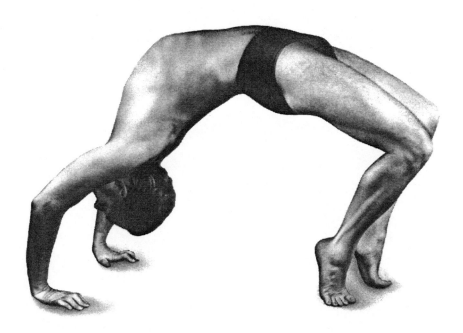

Chakrasana
THE CIRCLE POSE

Although the position of the body in this pose is similar to that in *Dhanurasana*, the Bow Pose, there are certain distinct differences. The backward bend in the Circle Pose involves the entire spine and neck, rather than only the lower back. The backward bend of the neck offsets any discomfort that may have come from the extreme forward bend of *Halasana*, the Plow Pose, and *Sarvangasana*, the Shoulderstand.

The general invigorating effect of this posture makes it one of the most important of all the *asanas*. It is an excellent posture to practice after the Plow Pose or the Shoulderstand if these poses have given you a cramped neck.

Psychologically, the Circle Pose is marvelous for recharging the body and mind with energy. It is a good pose to do in the morning upon awakening or whenever one feels tired or sluggish during the day. *Chakrasana* is said to be an antidote to obesity. *A word of caution:* Menstruating women should use caution during the first days of menstruation. It should not be practiced by women during pregnancy, or for several months after childbirth. In addition, people who suffer from hernia, "hollow back," or slipped vertebrae should avoid it.

TECHNIQUE

○ Lie on your back. Bring your feet up to the buttocks and place your hands, palms down, on the floor above the shoulders, with the fingers pointing toward the body.

○ Lift the body off the floor by straightening your arms and legs, relax the head back, and arch the spine as far up as is comfortable. *Note:* Relax the trunk as much as possible and be aware of the energy in the spine rather than of the tension in the body.

○ Feel that you are lifting yourself determinedly out of the long sleep of delusion, sluggishness, weakness, and apathy. Affirm mentally, "I am awake! Energetic! Enthusiastic!"

O Hold this position for not more than 15 seconds to start with, gradually increasing with practice to one minute.

O Return slowly to the floor. You may find it easier if you first lower your body to rest on the top of your head and let the rest of the body follow. *Note:* Never collapse out of a yoga position. Always be in full command of your body's movements.

O Rest in *Savasana,* the Corpse Pose (page 55).

O *Note:* The beginner may have difficulty assuming this position. Some of its benefits may be attained by simply bending backward over the seat of an armless chair.

An alternative method of getting into *Chakrasana* is as follows:

O Lie on your back. Bring your feet up to the buttocks and place your hands, palms down, on the floor above the shoulders, with the fingers pointing toward the body.

O Lift the trunk, supporting your weight on the feet and shoulders. The neck and head remain on the floor.

O Raise your body, supporting the weight on the feet, hands, and top of the head, with as much of the weight as possible forward on the feet.

O Lift the body completely, with your head relaxed backward, arms straightened, and the body supported entirely on the arms and legs.

○ To come out of the pose, reverse the preceding four steps slowly.

○ Adepts may prefer to bend backward from a standing position, their hands over their heads, until their hands touch the ground. To learn this method of assuming the Circle Pose, you may stand with your back to a wall and "walk" down the wall with your hands. The closer the hands can be brought to the feet, the more perfect the pose.

*"Come join me, friends,
and share my feast of joy!"*

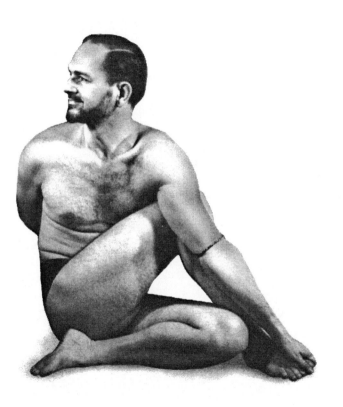

Ardha-Matsyendrasana
THE HALF SPINAL TWIST

This is one of only two postures that I know have been named after great yogis. Matsyendra lived in ancient times. His Full Spinal Twist is almost impossible for the average person to perform, but the Half Spinal Twist is not difficult for most people.

Physically, the Half Spinal Twist adjusts the vertebrae and exercises the spine, making it more limber. This posture is also good for constipation and for the sex organs. It beneficially stimulates all the trunk organs—the kidneys, liver, and spleen—and is good for a stiff or aching back.

Spiritually, if one can relax in this pose, he will feel that the energy is being forced up the spine into the region opposite the heart. This region, as everyone knows who has experienced a deep, sensitive love, is the center in the body from which feelings of love radiate. Yogis say that this dorsal center, or *anahat chakra*, needs to be stimulated, its rays of energy directed toward the brain. Divine love is thereby awakened. *Ardha-Matsyendrasana*, by forcing the energy up the spine to this region, helps to stimulate the *anahat chakra* and

awaken the feeling of love. The heart quality experienced in this twisted position, however, does not easily travel further upward toward the brain. Rather, its natural movement is outward. It may be felt to express itself as an outflow of compassion, rather than as devotion to God.

TECHNIQUE

○ Sit with your legs straight out before you. Draw your right foot toward you, bring it under the left leg, and place the foot to the left of your body, touching the left buttock.

○ Bend your left knee and place the left foot over the right knee, on the floor to the right of it.

○ Twist your body slowly to the left, placing the left hand on the floor briefly if necessary for balance. Then bring your right arm to the left of your upraised knee, locking the elbow on the outside of the knee. Now grasp your left foot with your right hand.

○ Bring the left arm as far as it will go around the back of your body at waist level, keeping the palm turned outward.

○ Turn your head to the left, but not so far as to strain the neck.

○ Sit as upright as you can. *Note:* If your muscles are tensed in this position, hold it for a few seconds only, increasing the time gradually to a maximum of one minute. If you can relax in this pose, hold it for as long as it is comfortable.

○ If you have even the desire for enlightenment, you have already progressed far on the evolutional path.

Look back now to all those creatures who are less fortunate than you in their understanding of life's purpose. Sitting comfortably in this posture, call them, by the magnetic power of your love, to join in your search for lasting values. Affirm mentally, "Come join me, friends, and share my feast of joy!"

○ After coming slowly out of the pose, relax in an easy cross-legged sitting position or in the Hero's Pose: keep the right leg bent on the floor and place the left leg, knee bent, over the right leg, hands holding the feet.

○ Repeat the pose in the opposite direction. One twist in each direction will suffice.

"Come join me, friends,
and share my feast of joy!"

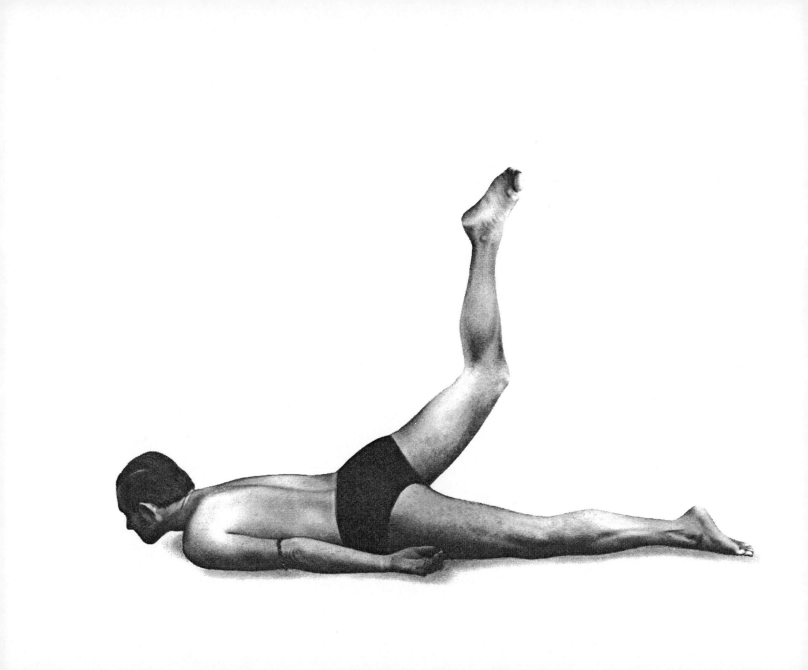

Ardha-Salabhasana
THE HALF LOCUST POSE

TECHNIQUE

○ Lie face down, with your arms at your sides.

○ Inhale and lift the left leg upward from the hip, keeping the leg as straight as possible and the hip on the floor.

○ Feel the energy being drawn from the feet and legs up into the base of the spine. Hold this position about 15 seconds to begin with, increasing it gradually to 30 seconds, or not more than one minute.

○ Repeat, lifting the right leg.

○ For an explanation as to why no affirmation accompanies this pose, see *Salabhasana*, the Full Locust Pose, which follows.

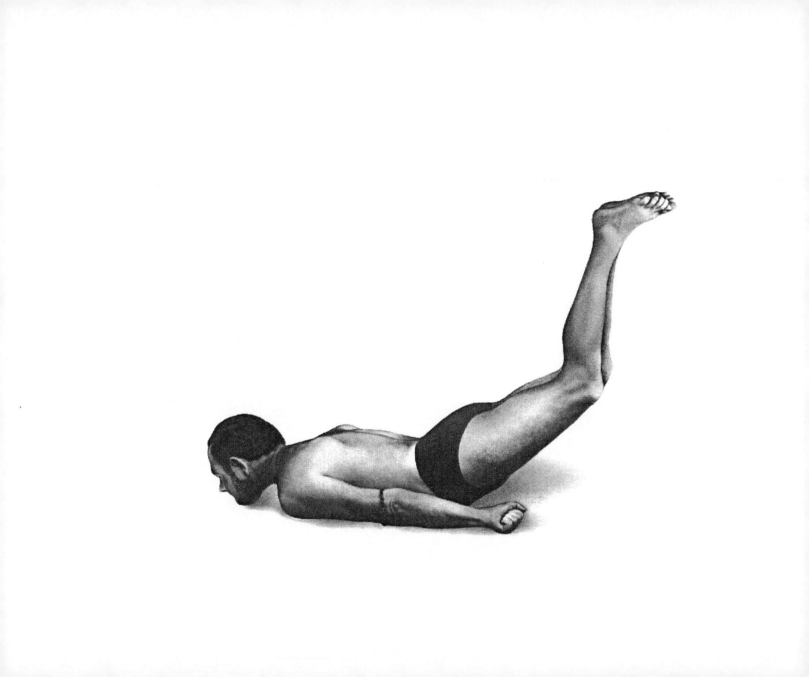

Salabhasana
THE FULL LOCUST POSE

Salabhasana is one of the most strenuous of the poses. It gives vigorous and beneficial exercise to the diaphragm and the heart muscles. It helps to strengthen the arms and back, and promotes health in the nerves of the lower back and legs. Its deepest benefits, as in most of the yoga postures, are spiritual—the raising of the energy from the lower extremities of the body as a preparation for concentration and meditation.

TECHNIQUE

O Lie face down, with your arms at your sides, as in *Ardha-Salabhasana.*

O Clench your fists with the palms turned upward so that the backs of the hands press against the floor. Rest the chin on the floor.

O Now inhale, then lift the lower body up with the strength of the arms, back, and legs to form a bow with the body in such a way that nothing below the navel remains touching the floor.

O Hold the breath as long as you hold the position itself. When you feel a need to breathe, exhale slowly and come down to a prone position.

O Repeat once or twice if you wish.

O While in the position, feel that all the energy is being drawn from the legs and focused at the base of the spine.

O It is difficult to make a mental affirmation in this strenuous position, but the energy that is brought into play can itself be used as a focal point for one's awareness.

"With shafts of will
I pierce the heart of worries."

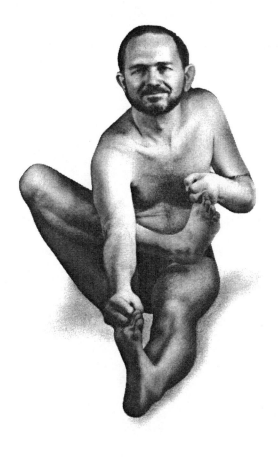

Akarshana Dhanurasana
THE PULLING-THE-BOW POSE

Akarshana Dhanurasana is excellent for promoting the overall vitality of the body. It also relieves chronic constipation and is good for the digestion. It is good for arthritis in the legs, knees and arms, and tends to remove fat from the middle part of the body.

TECHNIQUE

○ Sit with the legs outstretched before you.

○ Draw the left foot toward you, grasping it by the big toe with the fingers of the right hand, bringing it as close to your head as is comfortable.

○ Reach forward *over* the left leg with the left hand and grasp the big toe of the right foot, keeping the right leg straight. Affirm mentally, "With shafts of will I pierce the heart of worries."

○ Hold the pose for up to 30 seconds, gradually increasing the time to as long as six minutes.

○ Repeat with the opposite sides.

Inverted Poses

*H*aving released the energy, by means of the spinal stretching postures, to flow freely in the spine, it is now time to direct its flow upward, toward the brain. For this purpose, the inverted poses are marvellously effective.

In addition to the psychological and spiritual value, already discussed in this book, of directing the energy into the upper spine and the brain, there are great physical benefits to be derived from these inverted poses.

The body, in its usual upright position, is affected in only one direction by the earth's gravity: downward. As a result, the blood flows more to the lower extremities than to the brain. Toxins settle in the lower part of the abdomen, irritating the colon and the reproductive organs. Varicose veins and otherwise sore legs and feet are a common complaint, especially in the case of people whose work causes them to stand much of the time, and in people after middle age. Another evidence of the body's gradual surrender to the compelling force of gravity is a general sagging of the abdomen and of the abdominal organs, a condition all too common in middle age.

To help the body regain its natural balance is the physiological purpose of these inverted poses. Daily practice reduces varicose veins, hemorrhoids, unnatural sex hunger, * a sagging abdomen, and other disturbances of the lower body. On the plus side, these postures stimulate and rejuvenate the

glands and organs above the heart. They refresh the skin of the face, often making middle-aged persons look youthful again. The inverted poses stimulate the brain, thereby improving one's memory and powers of concentration, and sharpening his general awareness.

The inverted poses have their specific, as well as their general, benefits. It is preferable, therefore, that one practice all of them. But for those persons who find Sarvangasana, the Shoulderstand, and Sirshasana, the Headstand, too difficult, Viparita Karani, the Simple Inverted Pose, the simplest of the three, will bestow many of the benefits of the other two.

The inverted poses should not be practiced by persons with high blood pressure (over 150 mm of mercury in young adults, and over 180 mm in older persons), weak hearts, diabetes, chronic constipation, or with diseases of the ears, eyes, or sinus. Nor should these poses be practiced when the blood stream is infected, nor when it is impure—for example, as a result of long confinement in a closed room. A final caution: Don't practice these poses after doing strenuous physical exercise.

---

* Transmutation of the sexual energy into physical and mental energy is greatly facilitated by the inverted poses. An even more excellent technique for transmutation of this energy was discovered by the great yogi, Lahiri Mahasaya, the "grand" teacher, or paramguru, of Paramhansa Yogananda. It may be learned from Self-Realization Fellowship, 3880 San Rafael Avenue, Los Angeles, CA 90065.

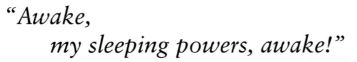

"Awake,
my sleeping powers, awake!"

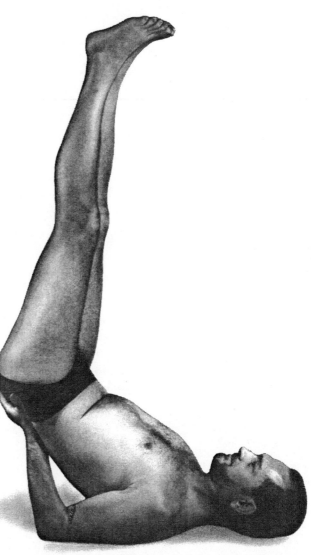

Viparita Karani
THE SIMPLE INVERTED POSE

The primary spiritual benefit of *Viparita Karani* is the stimulation of energy at the base of the spine. For the yogi, the awakening of this energy, known as *kundalini*, is of the greatest importance.

This position is also important for returning the body to a state of balance. Consider how much time you spend sitting or standing, thus allowing the blood to accumulate in the lower part of the body, pulled by the force of gravity. It is not only the blood; all parts of the body are affected by this gravitational pull. It is extremely important to your health and general well-being to counteract this pull by occasionally inverting the body.

TECHNIQUE

○ Lie flat on your back, arms at the sides, palms down. Inhale, exhale, press the small of the back to the floor, then raise your legs to a 45-degree angle and hold briefly. Now lift them to a 90-degree angle and again hold briefly.

○ Inhale, exhale, and using your hands for support, lift the hips from the floor.

○ Arch your lower spine so that the lower back is almost parallel to the floor. Use your hands for support by pressing the heels of the palms against the base of the spine, with the fingers spread out over the hips.

○ *Note:* Because considerable weight is placed upon the elbows when the hands are positioned so low on the back, many who practice this pose succumb to the temptation of bringing the hips a little higher and resting the hands in the middle back. Although this eases the pressure on the elbows, it misses the chief and unique purpose of this pose.

○ Concentrate on the pressure of your hands in the lower part of the spine, and feel by this pressure that you are awakening the energy in this area and causing it to flow up the spine toward the brain.

○ Affirm mentally, "Awake, my sleeping powers, awake!"

○ Hold this pose about 15 seconds to begin with, increasing the time gradually with practice to five minutes or longer.

○ Return slowly to a supine position and rest in *Savasana*, the Corpse Pose (page 55).

"Awake,
my sleeping powers, awake!"

*"God's peace
now floods my being."*

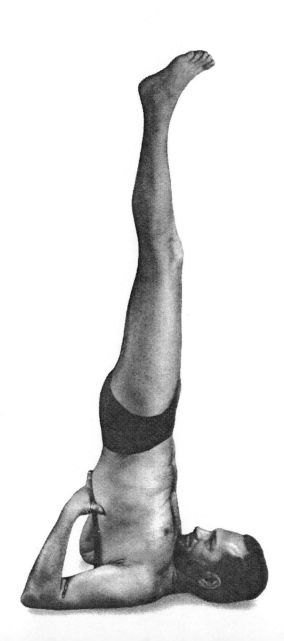

Sarvangasana
THE SHOULDERSTAND

The spiritual benefit of *Sarvangasana* is the deep calmness that ensues when the subtle energy of the body becomes concentrated in the cervical region. This pose, by stimulating that area, helps to induce calmness.

The Shoulderstand has been called the Whole Body Pose because of the gentle pressure exerted by the chin upon the thyroid gland, which regulates the body's metabolism. An additional benefit of this posture is the relaxing effect it has on the neck. *Sarvangasana* helps to relieve nervous tension and "tension headaches." The stretch in the back of the neck also stimulates the medulla oblongata. Because energy is distributed from this neural center to the whole body, stimulation of this center is another reason for the name, the Whole Body Pose.

TECHNIQUE

○ Lie flat on your back, arms at your sides and palms down. Inhale, exhale, then raise your legs to a 45-degree angle and hold briefly. Then lift them to a 90-degree angle and again hold briefly.

○ Inhale, exhale, press the small of the back to the floor, and using your hands to support your back, lift the hips slowly until the body is vertical, with the chin pressed firmly into the throat and the weight resting on the shoulders. The body should be in a straight line from feet to shoulders.

○ *Note:* It helps in this pose and in *Halasana*, the Plow Pose, to place a folded blanket under the shoulders with the folded edge directly in line with the shoulder line. This will take some of the pressure off the neck, while still allowing for a good stretch.

○ Continue to use your hands to support your back, but don't use them to hold up the body weight any more than necessary. Relax in this pose as well as you can.

○ Concentrate on the cervical region at the base of the neck. Feel that the energy in your body is becoming concentrated in that area.

○ Affirm mentally, "God's peace now floods my being."

○ Remain in *Sarvangasana* 30 seconds to start with. Increase the time gradually (but never beyond the point of comfort) to several minutes.

○ Return slowly to your original position and rest in *Savasana*, the Corpse Pose (page 55), for at least the amount of time spent in the Shoulderstand.

○ A good balance to *Sarvangasana* is *Matsyasana*, the Fish Pose (page 53).

*"God's peace
now floods my being."*

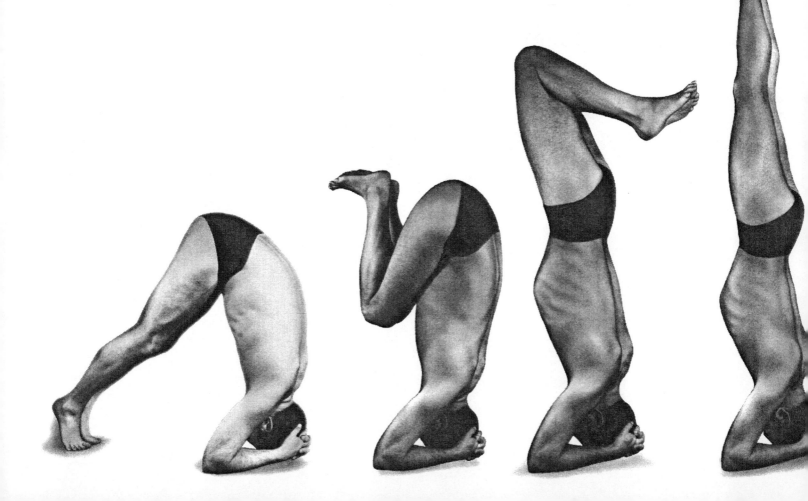

"I am He! I am He!
        Blissful Spirit, I am He!"

Sirshasana
THE HEADSTAND

The Headstand is one of the most important, but, alas for many people, one of the most difficult poses to practice. Because of its difficulty, many students make the mistake of trying to kick themselves up into it, as if it were an exercise in gymnastics—a procedure that, as often as not, lands them flat on their backs! Unless one assumes this pose slowly and with complete control, he may injure his neck. It is more important in this pose than in most to "make haste slowly."

A compromise with perfection may be necessary to start with. You may use the help of a wall, or better still, of a corner of your exercise room. This prop will give you the confidence gradually to stand on your own. You may also, while learning the pose, make use of the "tripod" position that is common to Western gymnastics, putting the hands on the floor in such a way as to form a tripod with your head. Until you can assume *Sirshasana* properly, however, you will not be able to relax while standing on your head; thus you will miss the fullest benefits of this position.

You have directed the energy upward from the base of the spine in *Viparita Karani*, the Simple Inverted Pose. By *Sarvangasana*, the Shoulderstand, you have concentrated this energy in the cervical region. Now in *Sirshasana* feel the energy becoming centered finally in the frontal lobe of your brain.

Physiologists tell us that this is the most advanced part of the brain. It is this region from which we derive, or in which are centered, the higher aspects of our nature—conscience, reasoning power, and ideals. Yogis say that concentration on this area (especially at the point between the eyebrows) develops spiritual insight and leads to final enlightenment.

Cautions: In addition to the cautions sounded earlier for inverted poses in general, students will be well advised not to practice *Sirshasana* if they are too heavy or if their necks are weak, or if they have high blood pressure or heart disease.

TECHNIQUE

○ Kneel on the floor. Interlace fingers, and place the hands and elbows firmly on the floor, forming a right angle. *Note:* It is important not to spread the elbows too far apart; their support is essential for lifting you into the position.

○ Rest the forehead on the ground at the hairline, placing the back of your head between your hands. Then lift the knees from the floor.

○ Push upward with your hands. Then lift the knees from the floor.

○ Push upward with the legs, walking the feet slowly forward until the trunk reaches a vertical position, preferably with the back arched slightly backward.

○ You should now be able, with the help of your elbows, simply to lift your body off the ground. Keep the knees folded against the abdomen, with the feet up to the buttocks. When you are balanced comfortably in this position, proceed to the next step.

○ Raise the knees, keeping the legs bent, until your thighs form a straight line with the trunk. Thrust the hips forward to be in line with the thighs and trunk; otherwise you may fall over backward.

○ Finally, straighten your legs.

○ Once the body can be held perfectly vertical you will find it easy to relax in this position. Concentrate on the pressure of your weight on the forehead. Having brought the energy up the spine,

now concentrate it at the point between the
eyebrows and at the frontal lobe of the brain.

O Affirm mentally, "I am He! I am He! Blissful Spirit,
I am He!"

O After a minute or longer, return very slowly, in
reverse order, to a kneeling position. Rest
momentarily.

O *Note:* The duration of the pose should be one
minute to start with. It may be increased gradually
to several minutes.

O Then stretch out in *Savasana*, the Corpse Pose
(page 55), and go into deep relaxation.

Sitting Poses

The sitting poses are primarily for the purpose of meditation. It is not necessary to meditate in any of these positions, but it is helpful to do so. The classic meditation postures exert a beneficial pressure on certain nerves, helping to induce physical and mental steadiness. To sit with the feet turned upward, close to the body, makes it easier to raise one's energy and consciousness. The primary purpose of hatha yoga is to prepare body and mind for meditation. Having completed the foregoing series of postures—having, that is, swept out and cleaned your inner temple—sit in your temple now and worship.

Never force your legs into any of the sitting postures. Mastery should come gradually, even though it require months, or years, of practice.

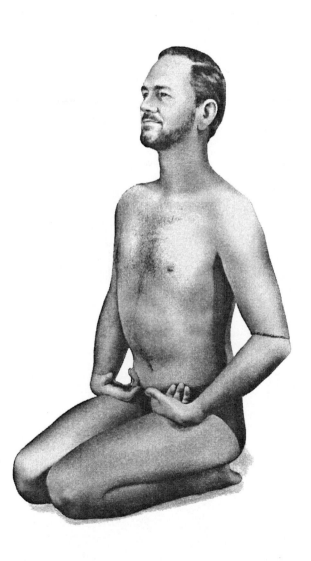

"*My mind is firm
and steadfast as a rock.*"

Vajrasana
THE FIRM POSE

Vajra means, among other things, "firm, hard, adamantine." In meditation, one is taught to attain a state of physical steadiness by one of two means, contradictory in approach, but not in effect. One may visualize the body as infinitely light—as composed of nothing but air or space. Having no body to move, one finds his mind soaring to loftier identifications. The other method is to imagine the body to be infinitely heavy, rock-like, and firm. Having a body that is too heavy and solid to move, the mind in this thought also finds that it is drawn to function on levels higher than physical.

The Firm Pose is ideal for this second practice. The pressure of the upper body upon the calves suggests to the mind a state of heaviness and solidity. Think of your body as being so firm that you cannot move a single muscle. Breathe normally and with every exhalation feel as if you were sinking downward into the floor. Gradually you will become aware of subtle energies in the body that move freely even though the body is still; you will begin to identify yourself with those energies, and with your own inner freedom from the body, rather than with the body itself.

Vajrasana is an excellent pose for attaining stability of mind. It is good, also, for flushing blood out of the lower legs. It is said to be good for the stomach, possibly because of the increase of blood to the abdomen after it has been pressed partly out of the legs, but more probably because of the sympathetic relationship that exists between the nerve endings in the feet and the different parts of the body. The middle part of the foot (around the instep) is said to be connected with the visceral organs. The ancient yogis no doubt found that the relaxation this pose gives to the instep exerts a beneficial stimulus to the stomach region.

Relaxing the feet relaxes the whole body. The simple feeling of relaxation in the feet in this position is indeed one of its happiest benefits, particularly if you concentrate on and enjoy this sensation. Try mentally to extend this relaxation upward into the whole body.

TECHNIQUE

○ Kneel on the ground with the feet stretched out behind you and pointed inward, so that the big toe of the right foot overlaps the big toe of the left foot.

○ Squat down until your buttocks rest on the inner soles of the feet. *Note:* You may support the body with the hands while assuming this position.

○ Cup the hands over the knees, or place the hands palms upward on the thighs, at the junction of the abdomen. You may also place the palms upward on the thighs, with the right hand resting over the left hand, thumbs touching.

○ Sit erect. Affirm mentally, "My mind is firm and steadfast as a rock."

○ *Note:* If you have difficulty getting into this pose, the following suggestions may prove helpful:

1. Assume an inverted pose first, to reduce the amount of blood in the legs.

2. Spread the knees apart slightly.

3. Push the calves outward to make it easier to rest your buttocks on the feet.

4. Raise and lower yourself several times on the knees to make them more supple.

5. Place a pillow under the ankles, or between the feet and buttocks.

6. Massage the knees and ankles with oil.

"My mind is firm
*   and steadfast as a rock."*

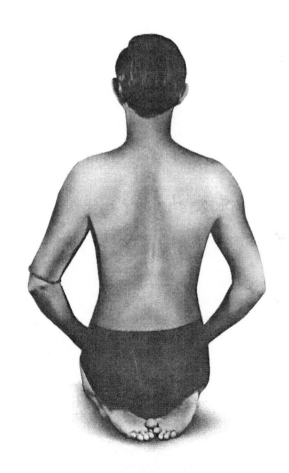

"I set ablaze the fire of inner joy."

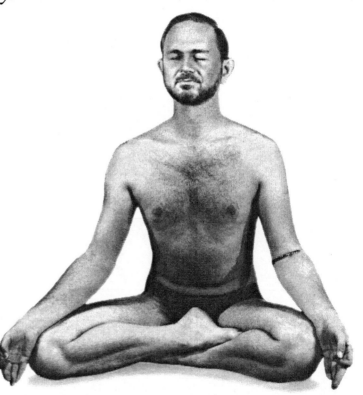

Siddhasana
THE PERFECT POSE

The name of this posture suggests that it is the pose for illumined beings (*siddhas*). To more practical purpose, however, it might be better translated, "The Pose for Attaining Perfection (*siddhi*)." *Siddhasana* is one of the two most important meditation postures, the other one being *Padmasana*, the Lotus Pose.

Siddhasana is so called for its influence upon the spinal centers, the awakening of which helps the yogi to develop *siddhis*, or yogic powers, and above all to become a *siddha*, or perfect being.

Be conscious of the spine in this technique. Draw the energy upward and focus it at the point between the eyebrows. After 20 minutes or so in this position, you will be surprised to see what a calming influence it has upon your body and mind.

This pose is said to be more beneficial for men than for women, although it may be practiced to great advantage by either sex. The locked position of the feet, even for women, sends energy from the lower extremities to the base of the spine, in a sense pushing the energy upward from the lower regions toward the brain. The position of the hands, similarly, suggests an inward drawing of the energy from those extremities to the spine.

TECHNIQUE

○ The Perfect Pose is practiced by sitting on a blanket in such a way that the feet are pressed in toward the base of the spine.

○ Sit with legs outstretched. Draw the left foot toward you and place the heel against the perineum, the space just below the reproductive organs. The sole should rest against the right thigh.

○ Now draw the right foot toward you, placing the heel against the pubic bone above the reproductive organs. Place it in such a way that the right heel is aligned directly above the left.

○ Men should place the heel above the genitals, preferably pushing the male organ inward upon itself so as to lock the genitals firmly between the heels.

○ To practice this pose to perfection, insert the toes of the right foot between the calf and the thigh of the left leg, and draw the toes of the left foot upward between the calf and the thigh of the right leg.

○ *Note:* If you cannot practice *Siddhasana* perfectly, bring the feet as close to the proper position as possible, even placing the right foot on the floor in front of the left, instead of above it in a position known as *Ardha-Siddhasana,* the Half-Perfect Pose—an engaging name! If keeping the spine straight in this position requires too much tension in the back, place a small cushion firmly under your buttocks to tilt the pelvis slightly forward.

○ One may place his arms and hands in any of several meditative positions, but in *Siddhasana* the classical position is to sit with the hands resting palms upward on the knees, the thumbs and forefingers joined lightly together, the remaining fingers extended comfortably outward from the palms.

○ This manual position is known as a meditative *mudra,* the purpose of a *mudra* being to make one conscious of the inward movement of subtle energy. In keeping with the purpose of *Siddhasana,* this *mudra* facilitates the withdrawal of energy and consciousness into itself.

○ Sit upright. Be very relaxed. Feel that the energy is being withdrawn up the extended fingers into the arms; up the arms into the spine. And feel that the energy at the base of your spine is being reinforced by the pressure of your feet against the crotch. Draw this energy upward, and feel that your whole being is becoming calmly, deeply centered at the point between the eyebrows.

○ Affirm mentally, "I set ablaze the fire of inner joy."

○ Remain in this pose as long as you like. In fact, yogis say that, to develop *nishta* (steadfastness), one should sit in this pose a little longer than one likes! That is to say, sit a little *beyond* the point of comfort.

"I sit serene, uplifted in Thy light."

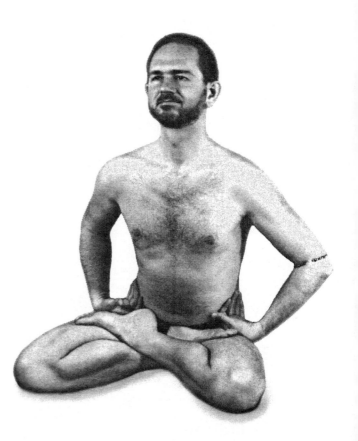

Padmasana
THE LOTUS POSE

Of all the yoga postures, this one is the best known, and—for many people—the most difficult. It is the most stable of the meditation poses. Its stabilizing effect, coupled with the upturned position of the feet, is, if anything, more helpful than *Siddhasana*, the Perfect Pose, in raising the bodily energy toward the brain. Everything about this position of the body suggests a natural rising upward of one's physical energies along with the upward soaring of the spirit within.

Padmasana is the classical meditative posture of the raja yogi (one who practices the ancient yoga science of meditation) while *Siddhasana* is that of the hatha yogi. The reason for this distinction is a basic difference in the approaches of these two yogic sciences. Hatha yoga might be said to assist the raising of the bodily energy by pushing it up from below. Raja yoga helps one to draw the energy up from above. We have already seen that these two approaches do not conflict; rather they complement one another. Hatha yoga is, in fact, the physical branch of the science of raja yoga.

It is vitally important, however, that this point be understood in its deeper implications. For if force is used, especially when there is no corresponding mental upliftment, serious psychic difficulties may result. This is a basic reason why the hatha yogi is counseled *never* to use force, and to approach his practice of the postures as much as possible with an uplifted state of consciousness.

As for whether one should use *Padmasana* or *Siddhasana*, he may be guided by personal preference.

Regular practice has been known gradually to accomplish the seemingly impossible. But remember always, in this posture above all: "Make haste slowly!"

Cautions: It is important *never* to force the legs into *Padmasana*. One may injure the knees if he does not stretch them gradually, even for a period of months.

Limbering exercises for Padmasana: Certain poses may help to prepare the body more easily to assume the sitting poses:

○ *Vajrasana*, the Firm Pose (page 115), helps to limber the knees, the ankles, and the feet.

○ *Janushirasana*, the Head-to-the-Knee Pose (page 65), helps to stretch the tendons under the knees.

○ *Paschimotanasana*, the Posterior Stretching Pose (page 61), helps to loosen the tendons under the knees and to stretch the pelvis, which makes it easier to sit straight in any of the sitting poses.

○ The inverted poses help to draw an excess of blood out of the legs, making it easier to arrange them into the more difficult sitting positions.

○ The Butterfly helps to prepare one for *Padmasana*—sit on the floor with the soles of the feet together, knees out. Gradually try to lower the knees and thighs to the floor.

○ Massaging the feet and ankles with oil can make them more limber.

○ The best limbering exercise of all, however, once you can assume any of these sitting poses, is simply to sit in it. After a minute or two, as one's legs relax into the position, one finds most or all of the initial discomfort disappearing.

TECHNIQUE

○ Sit on the floor on a blanket with your legs outstretched before you. Bring the right foot gently toward the body, and place it on the left thigh as close as possible to the abdomen. Then lower the right knee to the ground.

○ Now bring the left foot gently toward you, and place it as close as possible to the abdomen on the right thigh.

○ Sit erect. Affirm mentally, "I sit serene, uplifted in Thy light."

○ *Note:* The hands may be placed in a variety of positions. You may rest them palms upward between the feet, the right hand over the left. The palms may also be joined, with the fingers interlocked. Some yogis sit with the palms turned upward on the knees, or on the thighs, or set in closer to the junction of the abdomen. The important thing is to sit still and relaxed, with the spine straight.

○ Relax your body, and meditate calmly at the point between the eyebrows.

○ *Note:* If you find the Lotus Pose difficult, but desire earnestly to master it, you may find it helpful to place a pillow under the ankles to give them a little support, and to keep them from bending at an unnatural angle. A pillow under the knees, if they cannot be brought down to touch the floor, is also beneficial for the beginner.

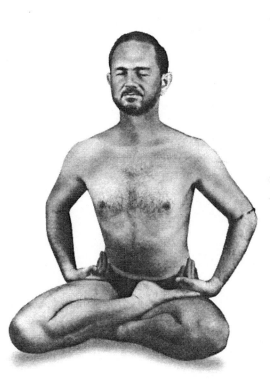

"I am Thine; receive me."

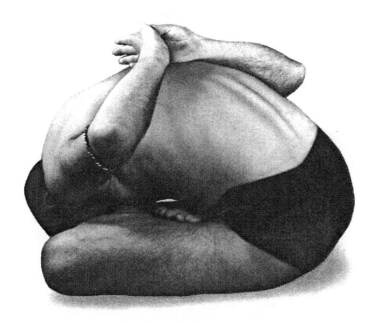

Yoga Mudra
THE SYMBOL OF YOGA

Yoga Mudra is usually translated to mean "The Symbol of Yoga." It is indeed this, for in all yoga practice, self-effort (which is implicit in the deliberate assumption of the yoga postures) must be combined with loving surrender to the Infinite Power, God. Man's self-effort must be done with a view, not to conquering the divine heights by human power alone, but to opening his consciousness so that God's light may reach down to him.

This posture, according to yoga tradition, helps to develop humility. The student may ask himself: Were the ancient yogis merely "milking" this pose for any conceivable benefits they might draw out of it? Any servile posture, any stoop forward, might as well be said to help develop humility.

Much more, however, is implied in this particular pose. Paramhansa Yogananda explained that ego-consciousness is centered in the medulla oblongata at the base of the brain. The disdainful angle of a proud person's head is due to tension, ego-induced, in this medullary region. Notice, the next time that you accept someone's flattery, how your energy gathers at the back of the head. Worldly man is ego-centered. Most of his thoughts and activities emanate from, or are in some way connected with, this medullary center. The aspiring yogi should strive always to release his energy from this point, and to center it in the Christ Center between the eyebrows. The medulla oblongata represents the negative phase of the brain's function; the point between the eyebrows, the positive phase. Both these locations are, in fact, the two poles of the same center.

The pressure of the forehead on the floor encourages the redirection of one's consciousness to the frontal region. The joining of the palms helps, finally, to induce an attitude of reverent worship.

Yoga Mudra takes the weight off the back of the neck, helping to reduce tension in that region.

TECHNIQUE

○ Sit in *Padmasana*, the Lotus Pose (page 123). Simpler crosslegged positions are permissible, but less desirable.

○ Lean forward until the forehead rests on the ground.

○ Bring your palms together behind you between the shoulder blades, pointing the fingers upward or, if you cannot do that, simply hold one wrist behind you with the other hand at the level of the waistline.

○ Pray mentally, "I am Thine; receive me."

"I am Thine; receive me."

3

Meditation

If a housewife spends all her time sweeping, dusting, and cleaning her home, what time can remain for her to sit down and enjoy it? Similarly, if all of the time that you can devote daily to your yoga practice is limited to practicing the physical postures, what time will remain for you to deeply feel and enjoy their benefits? A deep inner sense of enjoyment is, indeed, one of the benefits.

That is one important reason why relaxation between the postures is so repeatedly stressed. And that, too, is why their practice should be followed by at least 15 minutes of meditation.

What Is Meditation?

Meditation is not, as so many people assume it to be, a process of "thinking things over." Rather, it is making the mind completely receptive to reality. It is stilling the thought processes—those restless ripples that bob on the surface of the mind—so that truth, like the moon, may be clearly reflected there. It is listening to God, to Universal Reality, for a change, instead of doing all the talking and "computing" oneself.

Hints for Deeper Meditation

Don't put meditation in the "someday-when-I-find-the-time-for-it" category of your life. If you make it a point to meditate daily, you will soon see that the mental efficiency you derive from this practice will actually give you time to get all those other things done which now seem so difficult to squeeze into your busy schedule.

Try meditating every day for at least 15 minutes (half an hour would be even better). Usually the best time for meditation will be directly after your practice of the yoga postures. Yogis say that certain hours of the day are especially good for meditation: sunrise and sunset, when the sun's pull is at right angles to the pull of the earth on our bodies; noon, when the sun's pull opposes that of the earth; and midnight, when the two bodies pull together. These are said to be "rest points" in Nature, when the energy flow in our bodies is brought into temporary (if relative) balance. If you cannot meditate at these hours, to meditate at the same times every day is also desirable.

If you can set aside a room in your home as a little chapel and use it only for meditation, you will find in the course of only a few months that it will develop an atmosphere of peace which will help you to go deep when you sit to meditate.

Any comfortable sitting position will do, provided that the spine is kept straight and the body relaxed. There are several sitting poses that hatha yogis recommend, including *Vajrasana*, the Firm Pose, *Siddhasana*, the Perfect Pose, and *Padmasana*, the Lotus Pose. However, even a chair would be quite all right.

Place your hands, palms upward, on the thighs at the junction of the abdomen. Keep your chest up, but relaxed, and your shoulder blades drawn slightly together. Thus your body will resemble a bow, drawn into a position of spiritual readiness by the straight "string" of the spine.

Relax when you meditate. Don't strain. Everything in this world is done by straining—or so it seems to the worldly mind. But meditation comes only by deeper and deeper relaxation—physical, emotional, mental, and spiritual.

Breathing Exercise before Meditation

When you sit to meditate, begin by tensing the whole body, then throw the breath out and relax. Repeat two or three times.

Now inhale, counting mentally to 12; hold the breath, counting to 12; and exhale, counting to 12. Gradually, *if you can do so comfortably*, increase this count to 20-20-20, but keep the count equal for all three phases of breathing. Repeat this breathing exercise six to 12 times.

Your whole body should now be completely relaxed, and your mind ready for meditation.

A Meditation Exercise

Sit very straight and still. Think of your mind as a lake. At first, the ripples of thought may seem very important to you. That is because your awareness is centered in such a small section of your mental lake that even little ripples create a tumult. Gaze mentally outward in all directions; see how vast the lake really is. Mentally expand its shores farther and farther, until you realize how insignificant, in relation to its vastness, are the little thoughts that bob up and down here at the center.

Tell these thoughts to be still, to allow you to listen to the waves lapping on the distant shores of your mind. Then listen intently.

When everything is perfectly calm, feel on the still surface of your mind the soothing breath of Spirit. Do not be impatient. Allow the breezes of divine inspiration gently to caress you, to play over you as they will. Seek not to control them; remember, in nothing in life are you really the doer. Your ego is only an instrument.

Offer yourself wholly, ever more deeply and calmly, to the Divine.

May your daily practice of this ancient yoga science bring you increasing benefits of peace, physical and mental well-being, and inner soul-joy—the fruits of your ever-deepening Self-awareness!

4

Appendices

APPENDIX A

Breathing Exercises

What is Breath?

"And the Lord God formed man of the dust of the ground, and breathed into his nostrils the breath of life" (Genesis 2:7). Probably for as long as man has been on this fair planet the breath has been associated with life. At first glance, this association seems based merely on an obvious consideration; ordinarily, the quickest way to tell whether a person is alive (assuming the absence of voluntary movement) is simply to see whether he is breathing. Yet, the relation of breath to life has often been treated by wise men, including great yogis, as a deep mystery. Why? Life, of course, *is* a mystery, but it would seem to be reducing its magical aura almost to nonexistence to say that life is nothing but breath.

What is life? What do we mean, for example, when we say, "I feel so *alive* today?" Essentially, what we mean is that we have more *energy*. We instinctively identify life with energy, not with mere existence.

Then what is the breath? The body depends for its functioning on the intake of oxygen, and on the exhalation of waste matter in the form of carbon dioxide. But is the breath only a chemical? Not so, say the great yogis. They equate it with life, because they equate it with energy.

In India, in fact, one word, *prana*, is used for all three. For one thing, the breath is a valuable source of energy. Also, it acts as a strong stimulus to the natural energy-flow (or life-flow) in the body. Notice how, when you go to lift a heavy object, you always inhale first. Instinctively you understand that inhalation will help to bring you the strength you need for the work at hand. If you inhale energy consciously and deliberately while inhaling air, you will find that breathing is one of the prime means of drawing energy into the body.

Life, or energy, is more than the breath; nor is our understanding of life particularly enhanced by equating the two. But our understanding of the breath is greatly expanded by the association.

Proper breathing can help immensely to make you more "alive" and energetic. Begin from today to pay careful attention to your natural rhythms of breathing. You will soon discover in this seemingly simple life-function hidden spiritual treasures.

Breath and the Mind

When greeting a sunny day joyously, one tends to inhale, as if drawing into one's very lungs the wonders of creation. When you are excited, notice the rapidity of your breathing, and see how erratic its rhythms become. When one is ill or unhappy, he sighs as if to throw the burden out of his body or mind. When you are calm, see how that calmness reflects itself in a slow, harmonious rhythm of breathing. By gradually learning to breathe properly, you will be astonished to see how, simply through the breath, you can vitally change your mental outlook.

The breath, too, can be used in conjunction with mental affirmations to help one to develop courage, calmness, self-control, and other wholesome mental qualities. Affirmations can be made most effectively while the breath is held either in or out (though affirmation is generally considered most effective with the breath held out). When the breath is held still (either in or out of the body), the mind tends more easily to become steady, capable of entering deeply into whatever affirmation one has chosen to make. Exhalation, however, is associated with the surrender of the conscious mind—whether into sleep or into superconscious ecstasy. This is why it is generally considered best to make one's affirmations during the rest period following exhalation. It is also possible, however, to make a positive affirmation during inhalation and to feel with exhalation that one is casting out all weakness and negativity.

General Principles of Breathing

While doing yoga postures, it is a general principle to breathe in when the body comes up, whether into or out of any position, and to breathe out when the body goes down, either into or out of a position. For example, when coming up into *Chandrasana*, the Moon Pose, one should inhale; when coming out of it, one should exhale. One may breathe normally while holding the position. On the other hand, when going into *Trikonasana*, the Triangle Pose, which involves stooping, one exhales as one goes down into the pose, and inhales as he comes out of it. There are exceptions to this principle. In *Utkatasana*, the Chair Pose, for example, one inhales as he comes up, but holds the breath all the way down into the crouching position.

As a general principle (there are exceptions in some of the yogic breathing exercises), one should always inhale through the nostrils. The reasons for this principle are subtle as well as obvious. The obvious ones are that breathing through the nostrils filters out dust and impurities that otherwise would enter the lungs, and warms the air before it reaches the delicate inner membranes.

There is a further reason, not commonly considered, for nose breathing. The breath, as it comes up through the nasal passages, has a cooling effect upon the brain, refreshing it. "Keep cool" is an expression often heard when one wants to advise someone to remain calm. A cool nervous system is in a state of calmness and harmony. Heat is a sign of impurities, irritation, or imbalance in the flow of energy in the body and in the brain. Anger, for example, involving as it does a sudden and inharmonious increase of energy, has a heating effect upon the brain. Under the effect of anger, and of other "heating" emotions, it is difficult to think clearly.

It is important for the brain to "keep cool" if it is to function clearly and vigorously. Normally speaking, people who breathe habitually through the mouth tend to be somewhat dull-minded. Deep breathing through the nose, especially if it is done with a conscious effort to feel the coolness of the breath extending up into the brain, can actually stimulate the intelligence.

Most of the yoga breathing exercises are for this reason done through the nose. Certain exercises, however, involve inhalation through the mouth, though some even of these have as their ultimate aim the same as that of nasal inhalation, namely, the cooling of the brain and nervous system.

The general aim of hatha yoga is to use the body to push, or gently nudge, the energy upward toward the brain. There is a danger here, if one goes from gentle nudging to a brutal driving of the energy. This warning is particularly important in connection with the breathing exercises. One should not practice violent breathing exercises too long at a time. One should not practice too many breathing exercises at one sitting. When one feels nervous or emotionally upset, he should do only the most gentle of the breathing exercises. Finally, he should always be cognizant of the effects of these exercises upon his general nervous equilibrium. If they have an upsetting, rather than a calming, influence, they should be done for a shorter duration, or even abandoned altogether.

There are numerous breathing exercises in hatha yoga. It is by no means necessary, or even desirable, to practice all of them. To do one or two deeply is better than to skip eagerly through a long series of them. Indeed, one may well interfere with his progress by too great a variety of techniques.

A Simple Breathing Exercise for Energizing and Healing the Body

TECHNIQUE

○ Lie flat on your back in *Savasana*, the Corpse Pose (page 55). Let your arms rest at your sides, keeping the palms turned upward.

○ Inhale very slowly and deeply, and imagine that the breath is filling your feet. Feel the muscles, bones, and skin becoming permeated with the breath's energy until they fairly tingle with vitality. *Note:* Hold the breath only as long as you can do so comfortably, repeating the process, if you like, rather than over-extending the breath.

○ Do the same for the calves, the thighs, the hips, abdomen and stomach, hands, forearms, upper arms, chest, shoulders, back, neck, throat, jaw, tongue, facial muscles, eyes, brain—always slowly and gently, always with the deepest attention.

Double Breathing

This breathing technique can help to increase the inflow of energy into the body.

TECHNIQUE

- ◯ Inhale through the nostrils—a short breath, then a long.

- ◯ Exhale through the mouth and nose simultaneously—a short breath, then a long.

Alternate Breathing

This breathing exercise is used as a means of increasing your inner, spiritual awareness and for helping to balance and harmonize the currents in the spine.

TECHNIQUE

- ◯ Extend the thumb and the ring finger and the little finger of the right hand, closing the forefinger and middle finger against the palm.

- ◯ Close the right nostril with the right thumb.

- ◯ Inhale through the left nostril for a count of eight.

- ◯ Hold the breath, counting eight.

○ Lift the thumb and close the left nostril with the ring finger and the little finger.

○ Exhale through the right nostril to a count of eight. *Note:* A slight constriction in the throat, so as to make a gentle sound there during respiration, will help to increase the consciousness of the corresponding movement of energy in the spine.

○ Repeat six times.

Sitkari Pranayama

This is an excellent breathing exercise for making one more aware of the air and energy as it enters one's lungs, and also for developing the diaphragm.

TECHNIQUE

○ Put the tongue against the teeth.

○ Inhale forcibly through the mouth with a hissing sound.

○ Hold the breath in the lungs as long as you can do so comfortably.

○ Exhale through the nose, closing the lips, and feel the coolness of the breath penetrating up into the brain and spreading out into the entire nervous system. *Note:* Make the inhalation and exhalation equal in length.

Sitali Pranayama

The ultimate aim of this breathing exercise is the cooling of the brain and nervous system. It is said to be a good exercise to practice for cooling the body in warm weather. But remember, the mind plays the principle role in this technique, as in most others. Unless you use the imagination to feel the coolness of the breath extending soothingly through the nervous sytem, the automatic benefits of the technique will be insignificant. *Caution:* Do not practice this exercise more than six times at a stretch. Don't do it when the weather is very hot or very cold, nor on a full stomach, nor when unwell, tired, or excited.

TECHNIQUE

Note: To practice this you must be able to curl your tongue into the form of a tube. Some books teach one to stick the tongue far out in this exercise, but actually the tongue should be placed at the lips, not protruding beyond them. The rhythm of this breathing should be to a ratio of 1-4-2.

○ Inhale through the tube of your tongue and concentrate on the coolness that you feel at the back of the throat. *Note:* The inhalation should be gentle, not forced, so that most of the coolness is felt at the tip of the tongue, and the coolness at the back of the throat is caused not so much by the gush of air into the throat as by the extension of feeling from the tip of the tongue.

○ Hold the breath.

○ Exhale through the nose and feel this coolness spreading out into your nervous system, particularly up into the brain.

APPENDIX B

Poses and Affirmations

Akarshana Dhanurasana, the Pulling-the-Bow Pose
"With shafts of will I pierce the heart of worries."

Ardha-Matsyendrasana, the Half Spinal Twist
"Come join me, friends, and share my feast of joy!"

Ardha-Salabhasana, the Half Locust Pose

The Backward Bend
"I am free! I am free!"

Bhujangasana, the Cobra Pose
"I rise determinedly to meet all obstacles."
Or: *"I rise joyfully to meet each new opportunity."*

Chakrasana, the Circle Pose
"I am awake! Energetic! Enthusiastic!"

Chandrasana, the Moon Pose
"Strength and courage fill my body cells."

Dhanurasana, the Bow Pose
"I recall my scattered forces to recharge my spine."

Garudasana, the Twisted Pose
"At the center of life's storms I stand serene."

Halasana, the Plow Pose
"New life, new consciousness flow freely. See: They flood my brain!"

Janushirasana, the Head-to-the-Knee Pose
"Left and right and all around—life's harmonies are mine."

Karnapirasana, the Ear-Closing Pose
"My boat of life floats lightly on tides of peace."

Matsyasana, the Fish Pose
"My soul floats on waves of cosmic light."

Padahastasana, the Jacknife Pose
"What in this world can hold me?"

Padmasana, the Lotus Pose
"I sit serene, uplifted in Thy light."

Paschimotanasana, the Posterior Stretching Pose
"I am safe, I am sound. All good things come to me; they give me peace!"

Salabhasana, the Locust Pose

Sarvangasana, the Shoulderstand
"God's peace now floods my being."

Sasamgasana, the Hare Pose
"I am the master; all body energies are at my command!"

Savasana, the Corpse Pose
"Bones, muscles, movement I surrender now; anxiety, elation and depression, churning thoughts—all these I give into the hands of peace."

Siddhasana, the Perfect Pose
"I set ablaze the fire of inner joy."

Sirshasana, the Headstand
"I am He! I am He! Blissful Spirit, I am He!"

Supta-Vajrasana, the Supine Firm Pose
"Energetic movement or unmoving peace: The choice is mine alone! The choice is mine!"

Trikonasana, the Triangle Pose
"Energy and joy flood my body cells! Joy descends to me!"

Utkatasana, the Chair Pose
"My body is no burden; it is light as air."

Vajrasana, the Firm Pose
"My mind is firm and steadfast as a rock."

Viparita Karani, the Simple Inverted Pose
"Awake, my sleeping powers, awake!"

Vrikasana, the Tree Pose
"I am calm, I am poised."

Yoga Mudra, the Symbol of Yoga
"I am Thine; receive me."

Routines

Various sequences are given by different authors for the practice of the yoga postures. The sequences I recommend are based on the importance to hatha yoga practice of a peaceful and inward state of mind, and of the awareness and redirection upward to the brain of the energy in the body.

We begin with breathing exercises so that the postures may be done with the right attitude. Then we proceed with standing exercises, to help develop right posture and to center the consciousness in the spine. We then do various exercises to relax the extremities (the legs and arms)—for example, *Sasamgasana*, the Hare Pose, and *Supta-Vajrasana*, the Supine Firm Pose. We then concentrate on stretching and loosening the spine, with the purpose of creating a free and open channel for the energy to flow upward to the brain.

We then go into the inverted poses so as to use the force of gravity to draw this energy up the spine toward the brain. As we have said, the more the energy can be lifted up the spine into the brain, the more one is in a state of harmony and joy—the more, in short, he discovers the truth of the saying that the kingdom of heaven is within.

A long rest in *Savasana*, the Corpse Pose, follows after these exercises as a means of sinking deep into the inner awareness that has been awakened. After *Savasana*, one may assume any of the meditative poses and go into deep meditation.

Further rules regarding the sequences are primarily these: One should follow a bend in one direction with a bend in the opposite direction, so as always to return the body to a state of balance, even as the teaching of yoga is that one must neutralize the opposites of duality, and become identified with the one central reality, the adwaitic, or nondual Spirit which rests forever at the eye of the storm of creation. It is important, also, to rest after each pose, at least as long as one has held the pose, and longer if the heart has been so activated that it takes more time to return to its normal rhythm.

Normally, the body is more limber in the evening than in the morning. Morning practice of the postures can help you to wake up and face the day fully relaxed and at peace in yourself. Evening practice will help you to free yourself, physically and mentally, of the cares and tensions of the day. If you need a boost to your self-confidence, especially in the more difficult poses, do them in the evening when your body is more responsive. As a rule, the best time for doing the postures depends on personal choice. Most of them, however, should be done before meals, or on an empty stomach.

These routines are for the average person, who may have difficulty making time for more than a half hour to 40 minutes of practice at a time. Should you wish to devote more time to the postures, you may incorporate more of them, following the guidelines that I have just given. I suggest that if time is short, you might do different sets of postures on alternate occasions, either morning and evening, or on alternate days.

Always remember that it is better to do a few postures slowly and well than to do many of them hastily.

How to Begin Your Practice

If you can do the postures with a calm mind and with interiorized awareness, the benefit you derive from them will be vastly greater. Before practicing the postures, sit upright for awhile; do a few breathing exercises, then meditate at least a few moments. Above all, in your daily postures routine cast out of your body with every exhalation all laziness, hesitation, restlessness, and indifference.

Routine 1

TWENTY MINUTES

Practice *Vrikasana*, the Tree Pose—30 seconds on each leg. Rest 30 seconds after each practice.

Chandrasana, the Moon Pose—30 seconds each side. Rest.

Trikonasana, the Triangle Pose—30 seconds each side.

Utkatasana, the Chair Pose—30 seconds.

Lie down in *Savasana*, the Corpse Pose, for one or two minutes.

Paschimotanasana, the Posterior Stretching Pose—30 seconds, followed by another 30 seconds in *Savasana*.

Halasana, the Plow Pose—30 seconds in the final position.

Bhujangasana, the Cobra Pose—30 seconds:

Sasamgasana, the Hare Pose—30 seconds to one minute.

Rest in *Savasana* for two to five minutes.

Routine 2

THIRTY MINUTES

Sit cross-legged on the floor and inhale deeply, counting mentally to six; hold the breath for a count of six; exhale counting six; hold the breath out six counts. Repeat three times.

Practice *Sitkari Pranayama* six times, feeling the coolness of the exhalation permeating your entire nervous system.

Concentrate at the point between the eyebrows for two or three minutes. Stand up and do the Full Yogic Breath three times, extending your hands high above the head. Then practice the postures:

Vrikasana, the Tree Pose—30 seconds each side, with 30-second rests after each position.

Chandrasana, the Moon Pose—30 seconds each side, with 30-second rests.

Trikonasana, the Triangle Pose—same as above.

Utkatasana, the Chair Pose—30 seconds to one minute.

Padahastasana, the Jacknife Pose—30 seconds total time, followed by the Backward Bend.

Lie down in *Savasana*, the Corpse Pose, for two minutes.

Sasamgasana, the Hare Pose—one minute.

Janushirasana, the Head-to-the-Knee Pose—10 to 15 seconds each side with rests in between.

Paschimotanasana, the Posterior-Stretching Pose—30 seconds, followed by 30 seconds in *Savasana*.

Dhanurasana, the Bow Pose—15 seconds.

Bhujangasana, the Cobra Pose—30 seconds.

Lie on your back in *Savasana* and go into deep relaxation for five minutes.

Routine 3

THIRTY TO FORTY MINUTES

Sit cross-legged on the floor. Calm your body within and without. Practice Alternate Breathing (as learned in the preceding chapter) six times. Rest. Then practice *Sitkari Pranayama* three times. Inhale very slowly and deeply three times. Then sit calmly, concentrating your mind at the point between the eyebrows, until you feel completely centered in yourself.

Stand and practice the Full Yogic Breath three times, and Double Breathing (a short and a long inhalation through the nostrils, followed by a short and a long exhalation through the mouth and nose) three times. Then practice the following poses:

Vrikasana, the Tree Pose

Trikonasana, the Triangle Pose

Chandrasana, the Moon Pose

Padahastasana, the Jacknife Pose, followed by the Backward Bend

Savasana, the Corpse Pose

Janushirasana, the Head-to-the-Knee Pose

Paschimotanasana, the Posterior-Stretching Pose

Savasana, the Corpse Pose—30 seconds to one minute

Halasana, the Plow Pose, followed by

Karnapirasana, the Ear-Closing Pose—approximate total time, two minutes

Savasana, the Corpse Pose—15 seconds

Chakrasana, the Circle Pose—15 seconds

Ardha-Dhanurasana, the Pulling-the-Bow Pose

Bhujangasana, the Cobra Pose

End with *Savasana*, the Corpse Pose—approximately five minutes

Routine 4

FORTY-FIVE TO SIXTY MINUTES

Vrikasana, the Tree Pose

Garudasana, the Twisted Pose

Chandrasana, the Moon Pose

Padahastasana, the Jacknife Pose

Savasana, the Corpse Pose

Sasamgasana, the Hare Pose

Supta-Vajrasana, the Supine Firm Pose

Savasana, the Corpse Pose

Paschimotanasana, the Posterior-Stretching Pose

Janushirasana, the Head-to-the-Knee Pose

Savasana, the Corpse Pose

Halasana, the Plow Pose

Karnapirasana, the Ear-Closing Pose

Bhujangasana, the Cobra Pose

Chakrasana, the Circle Pose

Dhanurasana, the Bow Pose (optional)

Savasana, the Corpse Pose

Ardha-Matsyendrasana, the Half Spinal Twist

Viparita Karani, the Simple Inverted Pose

Sarvangasana, the Shoulderstand

Savasana, the Corpse Pose

Sirshasana, the Headstand

Savasana, the Corpse Pose—lie in deep relaxation for five minutes.

Resources

Ananda World Brotherhood Village

Ananda World Brotherhood Village, founded in 1968, is one of the most successful intentional communities in the world. Several hundred people live together on 750 acres of land and work in harmonious cooperation developing spiritual models for work, the arts, interpersonal relationships and marriage, and child raising.

Ananda incorporates many aspects of public and private enterprise, including a school system, market, construction company, a jewelry and gem store and a publications and recordings business. The community also operates a retreat which offers a variety of programs throughout the year.

Ananda members are guided by the inspiration of Swami Kriyananda in following the teachings of Paramhansa Yogananda.

The Expanding Light

Ananda's guest facility, *The Expanding Light*, offers a varied, year-round schedule of classes and workshops. You may also come for a relaxed personal retreat and do it your way, participating in ongoing activities as much or as little as you wish. The beautiful serene mountain setting, supportive staff and delicious vegetarian food provide an ideal environment for a truly meaningful, spiritual vacation.

Programs offered at *The Expanding Light* include:

Ananda Yoga for Higher Awareness—You can take weekend or week-long intensives in the original Hatha Yoga, as taught in this book. Experienced instructors will give you individual attention at your own skill level, from beginning to advanced. Also offered, is the **Yoga Teacher Training Course**, a month long course that offers certification in hatha yoga instruction.

How to Meditate—Meditation is the key to Self-realization. In these weekend and week long intensives, you'll receive personal instruction in the basic meditation techniques taught by Paramhansa Yogananda and learn how to bring the benefits of meditation into every aspect of your life.

Kriya Preparation—Kriya Yoga is the highest technique of meditation taught by Paramhansa Yogananda. This course will help you prepare for initiation in this ancient and sacred science of Self-realization.

Other programs offered at *The Expanding Light* include courses on yoga philosophy, spiritualizing your daily life, relationships, healing, "Experience Ananda" weekends, and much more.

For more information, please write or call:
The Expanding Light
14618 Tyler Foote Road
Nevada City, CA 95959
(800) 346-5350 or (916) 292-3279

Ananda Course in Self-Realization

Ananda Church of Self-Realization offers you a complete and practical training program in yoga, meditation, diet, the fundamentals of the spiritual path, health and vitality, affirmations, and much more—all a part of one mutually-reinforcing whole to bring every aspect of your life into uplifted balance. The course includes 22 lesson booklets, 1 book, 13 audio tapes, and a variety of optional videos which will deepen your understanding and practice of Paramhansa Yogananda's teachings. It also prepares you for initiation into Kriya Yoga, Yogananda's most advanced technique. The course can be completed in as little as a year, or may be studied over a longer period, depending on your individual needs, and offers extensive training and deep insights for the new or experienced spiritual seeker.

Part 1: Lessons in Meditation

Learn the basic techniques of meditation through clear, step-by-step instructions. Experience the importance of the breath/mind connection and the power of the focused mind. Learn also Paramhansa Yogananda's Energization Exercises, a unique system of exercises for controlling and increasing your energy level and overcoming fatigue. This course offers techniques of the path of Kriya Yoga including the Hong-Sau technique of concentration. Includes an illustrated, lay-flat book and two cassette tapes or CDs with guided meditations, visualizations, and guided Energization exercises. $24.95

Part II: Art and Science of Raja Yoga

The Art and Science of Raja Yoga is the most comprehensive course on yoga and meditation offered today. It gives us the balanced and complete approach of raja yoga. The course is organized around seven topics-Philosophy, Meditation, Postures, Breathing, Routines, Healing Principles and Techniques, and Diet. It includes in-depth discussions of the paths of karma, bhakti, and gyana yoga. The author, Swami Kriyananda, excels in showing the interdependence of these seemingly separate areas and how all of them, when correctly approached, further our spiritual progress. Includes a CD: talk on meditation, guided Yoga Postures, and guided visualization. $24.95

Part III: The Path of Kriya Yoga

The Path of Kriya Yoga lessons include six lessons and four cassette tapes. They cover: Discipleship, the Aum Technique and Kriya Yoga preparation. The discipleship lessons give Swami Kriyananda's insights into the meaning and practice of discipleship and stories of his personal experiences with Paramhansa Yogananda. They help prepare the student for an at-home Discipleship Initiation. Discipleship Initiation is a requirement for Kriya Yoga Initiation.

After Discipleship Initiation, the student receives the second part of The Path of Kriya Yoga lessons: the AUM technique and Kriya Yoga preparation techniques. $49.95

Other titles available from Crystal Clarity Publishers

Autobiography of a Yogi

by Paramhansa Yogananda

One of the great spiritual classics of all time. This is a verbatim reprinting of the original 1946 edition. Although subsequent reprintings, reflecting revisions made after the author's death in 1952, have sold over a million copies and have been translated into more than 19 languages, the few thousand of the original have long since disappeared into the hands of collectors. Now the 1946 edition is again available, with all its inherent power, just as the great master of yoga first presented it.

Trade paper $14.00

Yoga Therapy for Menopause

by Lennie Martin, FNP & Barbara Bingham, PT

Tens of millions of women are currently experiencing menopause or pre- or post-menopausal symptoms. This book uses yoga as a comprehensive, permanent solution to standard treatments that are often laden with dangerous side effects. Yoga and related practices are used to help alleviate mood swings, hot flashes, brain fog, as well as a multitude of other symptoms. Routines and advice are simple, easy-to-understand, non-sectarian, and require no prior practice of yoga
Hardcover $14.00

Yoga Therapy for Overcoming Insomnia

by Peter Van Houten , MD & Gyandev McCord, PhD

Insomnia is one of the most common health complaints in America. This is the first book that uses yoga as a comprehensive, permanent alternative solution to standard, often only marginally effective, treatments that could be laden with dangerous side effects. Routines and advice are simple, easy-to-understand, succinct, non-sectarian, and require no prior knowledge or practice of yoga. Four-color photographic illustrations throughout, presented in a beautiful gift-book format.
Hardcover $14.00

Yoga Therapy for Headache Relief

by Peter Van Houten , MD & Gyandev McCord, PhD

Headaches are one of the most common and aggravating health problems we experience. More than 40 million Americans suffer from serious or chronic headaches sometime in their lives and consume over 30,000 TONS of over-the counter painkillers each year. Yoga Therapy for Headache Relief is the first book that uses yoga as a comprehensive, permanent alternative solution to the standard—often only marginally effective—treatments. Topics covered include: the different types of headaches and how to tell them apart; how yoga can help them; two safe, effective routines—one short, the other longer—detailing which yoga postures to use for best results and much more.
Trade Paper $14.00

Meditation for Starters

by J. Donald Walters

Meditation brings balance into our lives, providing an oasis of profound rest and renewal. Doctors are prescribing it for a variety of stress-related diseases. This award-winning book offers simple but powerful guidelines for attaining inner peace. Learn to prepare the body and mind for meditation, special breathing techniques, ways to focus and "let go," develop superconscious awareness, sharpen your willpower, and increase intuition and calmness. Meditation for Starters is available as a book & CD set and as a 79-minute video. Each item is also sold separately.
Trade Paper: $9.95

Book with companion CD: $19.95

Intuition for Starters

by J. Donald Walters

Every day we are confronted with difficult problems and thorny situations for which we either don't have enough information to make clear-cut decisions or for which there is no easy intellectual answer. At these moments, we all wish that there was another way to know how to make the right choice. Fortunately, there is another way: through using our intuition. More than just a "feeling" or a guess, true intuition is one of the most important—yet often least developed—of our human faculties.

Intuition for Starters will explain what true intuition is, where it comes from, the practices and attitudes necessary for developing it, and how to tap into intuitive guidance at will.
Trade Paper: $9.95

Charkras for Starters

by Savitri Simpaon

Long a popular subject in metaphysical and Eastern spirituality circles, interest in the chakras has recently crossed over into the consciousness of mainstream America. Yet, for all of the newfound interest, until now, there has yet to be written a concise, easy-to-read guide to this most intriguing of topics. In Chakras for Starters, Savitri Simpson demystifies and explains what chakras are, how to work with them, and the benefits accrued from doing so. Readers will learn how working with the chakras can help them feel a greater sense of security, self-control, heartfulness, centeredness, intuition, and spiritual transformation.
Trade Paper: $9.95

Vegetarian Cooking for Starters

by Diksha McCord

Interest in vegetarian eating has been exploding across the country over the last decade. Even many of those who may not want to eat a completely vegetarian diet now recognize that healthy living requires the incorporation of at least some vegetarian principles and foods into their diets. Yet many people are still confused by the many different theories, fads, and techniques championed by various proponents of healthy eating. In *Vegetarian Cooking for Starters,* Blanche McCord gives straightforward, easy-to-follow dietary advice, immediately useful explanations on how to prepare basic ingredients for cooking, and simple but delicious recipes that will quickly help readers incorporate vegetarian meals into their diet.
Trade Paper: $9.95

How To Meditate

by John (Jyotish) Novak

This handbook on meditation is an aid to calmness,

clarity of mind, and, ultimately, inner communion with God. It offers clear instruction on the basic preparation for meditation, how to quiet the mind and senses, and breathing techniques. Much loved by readers for its clarity, How To Meditate is written by a disciple of Yogananda who has been teaching and practicing meditation for 28 years.
Trade Paperback $7.95

Spoken Word

Chakras for Starters

This recording offers a clear explanation of what the chakras are and how they function. It also includes guided meditations and visualizations for each chakra, allowing the listener to quickly and easily access the healing power deep within. Each meditation is accompanied by the music of composer Donald Walters.
CD: $10.95   60 minutes

Metaphysical Meditations

These thirteen guided meditations, based on the mystical poetry of Paramhansa Yogananda, are ideal for evoking deep, spiritual awareness. Set to a background of well-known and inspiring classical music, Metaphysical Meditations draws listeners inward to the calm, joyful, expansive states of awareness that accompany deep meditation.
CD: $10.95   40 minutes

Music

The Mystic Harp

J. Donald Walters captures the haunting, mystical quality of traditional Celtic music on this richly orchestrated album of Celtic harp solos, performed by Derek Bell of the Chieftains.
CD: $15.95   70 minutes

Relax: Meditations for flute and cello

Listeners will be taken on a journey deep within, helping them to experience a dynamic sense of peace and calmness. Relax is specifically designed to slow respiration and heart rate, bringing listeners to their calm center. The recording features fifteen melodies on flute and cello, accompanied by harp, guitar, keyboard, and strings.

David Eby, cellist for the internationally renowned Pink Martini, joins the highly acclaimed flutist, Sharon Brooks, for their second collaboration together.

CD: $15.95   70 minutes

I, Omar

If the soul could sing, here would be its voice. I, Omar is inspired by The Rubaiyat of Omar Khayyam. Its beautiful melody is taken up in turn by English horn, oboe, flute, harp, guitar, cello, violin, and strings. The reflective quality of this album makes it a perfect companion for meditation, quiet reading or other inward activities.

CD: $15.95   60 minutes

Life Is the Quest for Joy

This exquisite instrumental reaches deep into the heart, producing a feeling of profound relaxation, and an inward, meditative awareness. One melody embraces the human condition: the love, hope, disappointment, and pain that human beings experience in the their quest for joy. A thrilling experience in music, and in consciousness.

CD: $15.95   69 minutes

Videos

Yoga for Busy People

The first yoga video designed especially for people short on time, but who would nonetheless want to experience all of the many benefits of hatha yoga. The three 25-minute routines work together to create a video usable any time of the day, in any circumstance.

DVD: $14.95   75 minutes

Yoga to Awaken the Chakras

One of the only videos of its kind, Yoga to Awaken the Chakras will help practitioners work with the subtle energies of the body. Postures, special exercises, and mini-meditations are discussed and demonstrated to help the practitioner develop an awareness of the chakras and their qualities.

DVD: $14.95   75 minutes

Yoga for Emotional Healing

Yoga postures are beneficial not only for stress reduction and well-being; they can also be powerful tools for healing harmful emotional states. This video teaches how to use yoga postures and related practices to overcome anxiety, anger, depression, hurt feelings, negativity, doubt, and a host of emotional imbalances.
DVD: $14.95   75 minutes

About the Author

New Directions magazine of Vancouver, B.C., describes Swami Kriyananda as "Perhaps the most respected non-Indian exponent of yoga in the world." He has devoted his life of discipleship to clarifying the ancient teachings of yoga for Western man. He is the founder of the world's most successful intentional community, Ananda World Brotherhood Village, near Nevada City, California, with branches in Sacramento and Mt. View, CA; Seattle, WA; Portland, OR; Dallas, TX; Assisi, Italy; and Delhi, India. There the principles of yoga guide the lives of the more than 1000 members.

Kriyananda brings an alternative to the intensively physical, achievement-oriented schools of yoga postures that are currently prevalent in the West. His approach is in the tradition of ancient Hatha Yoga and of his own guru, the great Indian master Paramhansa Yogananda, author of the widely read and respected book on yoga, *Autobiography of a Yogi*. Swami Kriyananda brings the yoga science back to its central focus as an integral part of the meditative science of Raja Yoga.
What is the true purpose of Hatha Yoga? Not only greater flexibility, radiant health, and other physical

benefits, but heightened awareness. Hatha Yoga, correctly understood and practiced, becomes an invaluable preparation for meditation, and can actually bring us into higher states of consciousness. Kriyananda brings a clear, logical mind, a down-to-earth common sense, and an ability to clarify difficult, abstruse truths to bear on the science of Hatha Yoga, and so guides the student into an experience of the spiritual center of the yoga postures.

Each pose is an expression of a particular, spiritually helpful and uplifting state of consciousness. As we learn to experience that state of consciousness within ourselves, to affirm its reality and to increase its strength and radiance within, we find our heightened awareness naturally reflecting itself in the outer positions of traditional Hatha Yoga. No longer imposing the postures on our bodies from without, we strengthen ourselves to the states of awareness from which the poses spring. An interplay between the physical, the mental, and the spiritual comes into effect. The bodily position suggests to the mind particular states of awareness, and these same states of awareness naturally express themselves in the position of the body.

From 1948, when he came to Paramhansa Yogananda and became his direct disciple, until Yogananda's passing in 1952, under Yogananda's direct supervision, Swami Kriyananda would often demonstrate for guests and visitors the Master's approach to yoga postures. After Yogananda's mahasamadhi (his conscious exit from the body), Kriyananda developed this aspect of his guru's teaching into the coherent system known as Ananda Yoga for Higher Awareness. In this book of the same name, in his home-study lessons, *Ananda Course in Self-Realization,* and in innumerable classes and seminars in India, in America, and in many other parts of the world, Kriyananda has brought this system to its flowering.